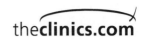

FOOT AND ANKLE CLINICS

Instability and Impingement Syndromes

GUEST EDITOR
Nicola Maffulli, MD, MS, PhD, FRCS (Orth)

CONSULTING EDITOR
Mark S. Myerson, MD

September 2006 • Volume 11 • Number 3

SAUNDERS

An Imprint of Elsevier, Inc.
PHILADELPHIA   LONDON   TORONTO   MONTREAL   SYDNEY   TOKYO

W.B. SAUNDERS COMPANY
A Division of Elsevier Inc.

1600 John F. Kennedy Blvd., Suite 1800, Philadelphia, PA 19103-2899

http://www.theclinics.com

FOOT AND ANKLE CLINICS Volume 11, Number 3
September 2006 ISSN 1083-7515
Editor: Debora Dellapena ISBN 1-4160-3805-1

Copyright © 2006 by Elsevier Inc. All rights reserved. No part of this publication may be reproduced or transmitted in any form or by any means, electronic or mechanical, including photocopy, recording, or any information retrieval system, without written permission from the Publisher.

Single photocopies of single articles may be made for personal use as allowed by national copyright laws. Permission of the publisher and payment of a fee is required for all other photocopying, including multiple or systematic copying, copying for advertising or promotional purposes, resale, and all forms of document de'ivery. Special rates are available for educational institutions that wish to make photocopies for nonprofit educational classroom use. Permissions may be sought directly from Elsevier's Rights Department in Philadelphia, PA, USA: phone: (+1) 215 239 3804, fax: (+1) 215 239 3805, e-mail: healthpermissions@elsevier.com. Requests may also be completed on-line via the Elsevier homepage (http://www.elsevier.com/locate/permissions). In the USA, users may clear permissions and make payments through the Copyright Clearance Center, Inc., 222 Rosewood Drive, Danvers, MA 01923, USA; phone: (978) 750-8400, fax: (978) 750-4744, and in the UK through the Copyright Licensing Agency Rapid Clearance Service (CLARCS), 90 Tottenham Court Road, London WIP 0LP, UK; phone (+44) 171 436 5931; fax: (+44) 171 436 3986. Other countries may have a local reprographic rights agency for payments.

Reprints. For copies of 100 or more of articles in this publication, please contact the Commercial Reprints Department, Elsevier Inc., 360 Park Avenue South, New York, New York 10010-1710. Tel.: (212) 633-3813; Fax: (212) 462-1935, e-mail: reprints@elsevier.com

The ideas and opinions expressed in *Foot and Ankle Clinics* do not necessarily reflect those of the Publisher. The Publisher does not assume any responsibility for any injury and/or damage to persons or property arising out of or related to any use of the material contained in this periodical. The reader is advised to check the appropriate medical literature and the product information currently provided by the manufacturer of each drug to be administered to verify the dosage, the method and duration of administration, or contraindications. It is the responsibility of the treating physician or other health care professional, relying on independent experience and knowledge of the patient, to determine drug dosages and the best treatment for the patient. Mention of any product in this issue should not be construed as endorsement by the contributors, editors, or the Publisher of the product or manufacturers' claims.

Foot and Ankle Clinics (ISSN 1083-7515) is published quarterly by Elsevier, Inc., 360 Park Avenue South, New York, NY 10010-1710. Months of issue are March, June, September, and December. Business and Editorial Offices: 1600 John F. Kennedy Blvd., Suite 1800, Philadelphia, PA 19103-2899. Customer Service Office: 6277 Sea Harbor Drive, Orlando, FL 32887-4800. Periodicals postage paid at New York, NY, and additional mailing offices. Subscription prices are $285.00 per year Institutional, $245.00 per year Institutional USA, $285.00 per year Institutional Canada, $230.00 per year Personal, $170.00 per year Personal USA, $190.00 per year Personal Canada, $110.00 per year Personal student, $85.00 per year Personal student USA, $110.00 per year Personal student Canada. To receive student/resident rate, orders must be accompanied by name of affiliated institution, date of term, and the *signature* of program/residency coordinator on institution letterhead. Orders will be billed at individual rate until proof of status is received. Foreign air speed delivery is included in all *Clinics* subscription prices. All prices are subject to change without notice. POSTMASTER: Send address changes to *Foot and Ankle Clinics*, Elsevier Periodicals Customer Service, 6277 Sea Harbor Drive, Orlando, FL 32887-4800. **Customer Service: 1-800-654-2452 (US). From outside of the US, call 1-407-345-1000.**

Printed in the United States of America.

CONSULTING EDITOR

MARK S. MYERSON, MD, President, American Orthopaedic Foot and Ankle Society; Director, The Institute for Foot and Ankle Reconstruction, Mercy Medical Center, Baltimore, Maryland

GUEST EDITOR

NICOLA MAFFULLI, MD, MS, PhD, FRCS (Orth), Department of Trauma and Orthopaedic Surgery, Keele University School of Medicine, North Staffordshire Hospital, Stoke-on-Trent, Staffordshire, England

CONTRIBUTORS

ADAM AJIS, BMEDSC (HONS PHYSIOL), MBCHB, MRCSED, Department of Trauma and Orthopaedic Surgery, Keele University School of Medicine, Stoke-on-Trent, Staffs, United Kingdom

DORY S. BOYER, MD, FRCSC, Foot and Ankle Fellow, British Columbia's Foot and Ankle Clinic, Vancouver, British Columbia, Canada

MURAT BOZKURT, MD, Associate Professor, Chief, 3rd Orthopedics and Traumatology Clinic, Diskapi Yildirim Beyazid Research and Education Hospital, Ankara, Turkey

JASON BROCKWELL, FRCSed(ORTH) , Orthopaedic Surgeon, Sports Physicians, Hong Kong

ALESSANDRO CAPRIO, MD, Paideia Hospital, Orthpaedic Unit, Rome, Italy

MAHMUT NEDIM DORAL, Professor, Department of Orthopedics and Traumatology, Hacettepe University, Faculty of Medicine, Sihhiye, Ankara, Turkey; Director, Department of Sports Medicine, Hacettepe University, Faculty of Medicine, Sihhiye, Ankara, Turkey

NORMAN ESPINOSA, MD, Fellow, Institute for Foot and Ankle Reconstruction, Mercy Medical Center, Baltimore, Maryland

NICHOLAS ANTONIO FERRAN, MBBS, MRCSEd, Department of Trauma and Orthopaedic Surgery, Keele University School of Medicine, Hartshill, Stoke-on-Trent, Staffordshire, United Kingdom

JAMES F. GRIFFITH, FRCR, Professor, Department of Diagnostic Radiology and Organ Imaging, Chinese University of Hong Kong, Shatin, Hong Kong

IFTACH HETSRONI, MD, Resident, Meir General Hospital, Sapir Medical Center, Kfar-Saba; Sackler School of Medicine, Tel Aviv University, Tel Aviv, Israel

BEAT HINTERMANN, MD, Associate Professor, Department of Orthopaedic Surgery, Chief, Orthopaedic Clinic, University of Basel, Kantonsspital Liestal, Liestal, Switzerland

ANISH R. KADAKIA, MD, Institute for Foot and Ankle Reconstruction, Mercy Medical Center, Baltimore, Maryland

JON KARLSSON, MD, PhD, Professor of Orthopaedics and Sports Traumatology, Department of Orthopaedics, The Sahlgrenska Academy at Göteborg University, Sahlgrenska University Hospital, Göteborg, Sweden

MARKUS KNUPP, MD, Senior Attending Resident, Department of Orthopaedic Surgery, Orthopaedic Clinic, University of Basel, Kantonsspital Liestal, Liestal, Switzerland

NICOLA MAFFULLI, MD, MS, PhD, FRCS (ORTH), Department of Trauma and Orthopaedic Surgery, Keele University School of Medicine, North Staffordshire Hospital, Stoke-on-Trent, Staffordshire, England

NIKOLAOS MALLIAROPOULOS, MD, MscSpMed, PhD, Director of the National Sports Injury Clinic, SEGAS, Thessaloniki, Greece

GIDEON MANN, MD, Professor, Department of Orthopaedic Surgery, Meir General Hospital, Sapir Medical Center, Kfar-Saba; Sackler School of Medicine, Tel Aviv University, Tel Aviv; The Ribstein Center for Research and Sports Medicine, Wingate Institute, Netanaya, Israel

DONALD J. MCBRIDE, FRCS, FRCS (ORTH AND TRAUMA), Consultant, Orthopaedic and Trauma Surgeon, University Hospital of North Staffordshire, Stoke-on-Trent, Staffordshire, United Kingdom

MARK S. MYERSON, MD, President, American Orthopaedic Foot and Ankle Society; Director, The Institute for Foot and Ankle Reconstruction, Mercy Medical Center, Baltimore, Maryland

MEIR NYSKA, MD, Professor, Department of Orthopaedic Surgery, Meir General Hospital, Sapir Medical Center, Kfar-Saba; Sackler School of Medicine, Tel Aviv University, Tel Aviv, Israel

FRANCESCO OLIVA, MD, University of Rome Tor Vergata, Faculty of Medicine and Surgery, Department of Orthopaedics and Traumatology, Rome, Italy

GEERT I. PAGENSTERT, MD, Senior Attending Resident, Department of Orthopaedic Surgery, Orthopaedic Clinic, University of Basel, Kantonsspital, Liestal, Switzerland

EMMANUEL PAPACOSTAS, MD, National Sports Injury Clinic, SEGAS, Thessaloniki, Greece

AGAPI PAPALADA, PT, National Sports Injury Clinic, SEGAS, Thessaloniki, Greece

CHANDRU RAMAMURTHY MRCS, DOrtho, Registrar, University Hospital of North Staffordshire, Stoke-on-Trent, Staffordshire, United Kingdom

MICHAEL SANCONE, MD, Department of Orthopaedics, Sahlgrenska University Hospital, Göteborg University, Göteborg, Sweden

JONATHAN P. SMEREK, MD, Fellow, Institute for Foot and Ankle Reconstruction, Mercy Medical Center, Baltimore, Maryland

FABIO TREIA, MD, S. Luca Hospital, Orthopaedic Unit, Rome, Italy

C. NIEK VAN DIJK, MD, PhD, Head of Orthopaedic Department, Academic Medical Center, University of Amsterdam, Amsterdam, The Netherlands

ALASTAIR S. E. YOUNGER, MB, ChB, ChM, MSc, Department of Orthopaedics, The University of British Columbia, Vancouver, Canada; Director, British Columbia's Foot and Ankle Clinic, Vancouver, British Columbia, Canada

CONTENTS

additional investigations, including cross-sectional imaging, and thoughtful interpretation of the information, one should rarely be caught out by misdiagnosis, multiple diagnoses, or unusual underlying causes.

We present a longitudinal observational study on classification of acute lateral ankle ligament injuries in track and field athletes, based on objective criteria. These very common and sometimes troublesome sports injuries are treated functionally, but there is a lack in international literature in predicting the time needed for full recovery. Taking into consideration (1) active range of motion, (2) edema, (3) stress radiographs findings, and (4) full rehabilitation time, we divided grade III sprains in IIIA and IIIB, proposing that these injuries can be classified in four categories (I, II, IIA, IIIB). The range of motion-edema-stress radiographs classification that we propose evaluates the severity of lateral ankle injuries, is an easy and practical method, and predicts full return in athletic activities without residual complaints, if the proper rehabilitation program is executed.

In 1975, Good and coworkers published a grading system that was based on four categories (excellent, good, fair, and poor) to evaluate the outcome of ankle injuries. Since then, at least six other scoring scales have been suggested to evaluate the success of conservative management protocols, assess the success of surgical procedures, or evaluate the severity and prognosis of an ankle sprain at the acute stage of injury. The most recent scoring system—probably the only one that was validated fully—was presented by Roos and coworkers. This article discusses various scoring systems that are used to evaluate this pathology.

Ligament injuries of the ankle are common, their management time-consuming and costly. The diagnosis and the early management of acute Grade I and II injuries is well codified. However, Grade III injuries have generated much controversy: early mobilization, cast immobilization, or surgery have all been advocated. One meta-analysis has shown marginally better results after surgical repair, but three Cohrane reviews have not been conclusive. The medium- to long-term prognosis is good to excellent in most patients regardless of the primary management regimen implemented. Nevertheless, several studies have reported residual symptoms, especially pain or recurrent instability in 10% to 30% of patients. Short-term prognosis is much improved with adequate acute phase management, such as compression pads, controlled range-of-motion training, and weight bearing or an Air-Stirrup brace. These studies have shown that absence from work can be shortened by approximately 50%, and return to sports by several weeks, without increasing the risk of residual symptoms. Many patients with residual symptoms after acute injury have prolonged peroneal reaction time, indicating proprioceptive deficit or muscular imbalance. Functional outcome after a well-supervised rehabilitation protocol is satisfactory in approximately 50% of these patients, even after several years of instability. Recently, prevention has gained increased attention, with proprioceptive training or external support, using either tape or brace. There is more evidence for bracing as a prophylactic measure. In patients with chronic symptoms, such as recurrent instability, secondary surgical procedures are successful in most cases. Anatomic ligament reconstructions produce satisfactory stability in most patients, are technically simple, and have a low complication rate.

intervention, the appropriate procedure should be selected according to their physical and lifestyle demands. The surgeon should gain familiarity with the full range of procedures, from open to percutaneous, and anatomic to nonanatomic. With proper patient selection, functional outcomes are excellent, with success rates from 80% to 90%.

Many techniques are available for surgical reconstruction of chronic lateral ankle instability. Nonanatomic procedures (or tenodesis procedures) cause numerous adverse effects, with restriction of motion of the subtalar and ankle joints and arthritis in up to 60% of patients. The procedures that use the tip of the fibula or the posterior aspect of the fibula for insertion of the calcaneofibular ligament are nonanatomic, and act as tenodesis procedures. Precise reconstruction of anatomy is the key to successful lateral ligament reconstruction. The plantaris tendon offers the opportunity to use local autograft tissue with high tensile strength, a long graft when harvested at the proximal calf, and without the further damage to the impaired lateral muscular control intrinsic in peroneal tendon harvesting.

Many techniques have been described for surgical management of lateral ankle instability. Anatomic repair and nonanatomic reconstruction have higher recurrence rates, and may be complicated by ankle stiffness. Anatomic reconstruction should be considered in stabilization for deficiencies of the lateral ankle ligament complex, as the initial construct is stronger while maintaining normal ankle mechanics.

The management of chronic lateral instability of the ankle remains controversial. In general, the anterior talofibular ligament (ATFL) must be reconstructed in all patients. Some will also need reconstruction of the calcaneofibular ligament (CFL) (or of its function) to regain stability of both the ankle and the subtalar joints, and to avoid recurrence of instability. After reconstruction, most authors report good to excellent results in 80% to 85% of patients. We describe an augmented reconstruction technique of ATFL and

CFL with a semitendinosus tendon allograft through a peroneal bone tunnel fixed with biodegradable anchors, and advocate this procedure as a safe, effective method to manage lateral ankle instability.

Many techniques have been described in acute and chronic lateral ligament insufficiency in the ankle. At present, the Brostrom-Gould and Chrisman-Snook procedures and their variations remain the "gold standard." Recent assessment of important etiologic factors has shed some light on the relationship between the original injury or injuries and the subsequent development of the varus tibiotalar joint with or without secondary osteoarthritis. The development of the Taylor Spatial Frame may well revolutionize its management. In the meantime, further consideration should be given to well-designed and evaluated randomized controlled trials, improved understanding of the biomechanics, and function of the ligaments; for example, proprioceptive function and their healing. Newer and less invasive arthroscopic and percutaneous techniques are being developed.

The medial ligaments of the ankle are injured more often than generally believed. Complete deltoid ligament tears are occasionally seen in association with lateral malleolar fractures or bimalleolar fractures. Chronic deltoid ligament insufficiency can be seen in several conditions, including posterior tibial tendon disorder, trauma- and sports-related deltoid disruptions, and valgus talar tilting in patients who have a history of triple arthrodesis or total ankle arthroplasty. This article focuses on the anatomy and function of the medial ligaments of the ankle and establishes a rationale for the diagnosis and treatment of incompetent deltoid ligament.

Both acute and chronic syndesmotic injuries can lead to significant morbidity. The key to management of acute injuries is anatomic reduction of the fibula and the syndesmosis. A high index of suspicion for syndesmotic injuries will allow the surgeon to avoid the difficult reconstruction options for chronic diastasis.

FORTHCOMING ISSUES

RECENT ISSUES

THE CLINICS ARE NOW AVAILABLE ONLINE!

http://www.theclinics.com

Foot Ankle Clin N Am
11 (2006) xv–xvi

FOOT AND
ANKLE CLINICS

Preface

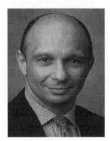

Nicola Maffulli, MD, MS, PhD, FRCS (Orth)
Guest Editor

This has been a great honor, and great fun! Instability of the ankle is a big set of words, and embraces much more than one would be led to think at first sight. Even words at times fail us, and one of the major things that I have been taught is that "laxity" is not the same as "instability." Indeed, one is a sign, the other a symptom, and the two do not necessarily have the same implications for patient management in clinical practice.

The articles in this issue arise from both the New and the Old World, and reflect the cutting edge practice of leaders in the field of ankle instability and impingement. Some concepts are well established, but are only chronologically "old": in reality, they have withstood the test of time, and we practice according to them. Other concepts are emerging, and with them new techniques. It is interesting to see what is happening. The use of arthroscopy has revolutionized the management of many ailments, and this applies to this field as well. The imaginative work of some pioneers will have great resonance, and will surely benefit our patients.

By our own nature, we orthopods are dazzled by biomechanics studies which, in reality, at times leave the bio- out of the biomechanics. Hence, mechanically stronger is not necessarily biologically better, as, in ankle instability, the work of Brostom showed 4 decades ago. Indeed, simpler and gentler may well be better for our ankles.

1083-7515/06/$ - see front matter © 2006 Elsevier Inc. All rights reserved.
doi:10.1016/j.fcl.2006.07.007

In the end, many thanks to all my authors: it has been hard work for them, but this issue has cemented friendships and produced new ones.

Nicola Maffulli, MD, MS, PhD, FRCS (Orth)
Department of Trauma and Orthopaedic Surgery
Keele University School of Medicine
North Staffordshire Hospital
Thornburrow Drive Hartshill
Stoke on Trent
Staffordshire ST4 7QB
United Kingdom

E-mail address: n.maffulli@keele.ac.uk

ELSEVIER
SAUNDERS

Foot Ankle Clin N Am
11 (2006) 451–463

FOOT AND
ANKLE CLINICS

Anatomic Factors and Biomechanics in Ankle Instability

Murat Bozkurt[a],*, Mahmut Nedim Doral[b,c]

[a]Orthopedics and Traumatology Clinic, Diskapi Yildirim Beyazid Research and Education
Hospital, Tirebolu sokak, Omrumce Apt., 27/18, Yukariayanci, Ankara 06550, Turkey
[b]Department of Orthopedics and Traumatology, Hacettepe University,
Faculty of Medicine, Sihhiye, Ankara 06100, Turkey
[c]Department of Sports Medicine, Hacettepe University, Faculty of Medicine, Sihhiye,
Ankara 06100, Turkey

Ankle sprains are common in both sport and leisure activities [1–14]. Despite the high success rates of conservative management, approximately 10% to 30% of patients develop chronic instability [7,15]. Surgery yields high success rates, but clinical problems such as functional or mechanical instability, persistent talar tilt, range of motion limitations, and pain may persist despite surgery [7,16]. In the studies on risk factors for ankle sprains, anatomic variations and biomechanical abnormalities come to the forefront [1–7,9,12,14]. The bone structure of the ankle and the surrounding ligaments interact in a complex mechanical fashion. The tibia plafond and fibula articulate with talus. The anterior talofibular ligament, the calcaneofibular ligament, the posterior talofibular ligament, and the deltoid ligament provide joint stability medially and laterally. In addition, the ligaments of the inferior tibiofibular joint and the talocalcaneal ligaments are supporting structures.

Bony anatomy of the ankle

The body of the talus is lodged in a deep recess formed by the lower end of the tibia and its medial malleolus, the lateral malleolus of the fibula, and the inferior transverse tibiofibular ligament. It contour is appreciated just distal to the anterior margin of the distal end of the tibia, which is palpable when the overlying tendons are relaxed. Despite its simple hinge-like appearance, usually in "uniaxial" style, the ankle has a dynamic axis of rotation,

* Corresponding author.
E-mail address: nmbozkurt@yahoo.com (M. Bozkurt).

1083-7515/06/$ - see front matter © 2006 Elsevier Inc. All rights reserved.
doi:10.1016/j.fcl.2006.06.001

shifting during dorsi- and plantar flexion [7,10–12,16–19]. The anterior, medial, posterior, lateral, and distal surfaces in the distal end of the tibia project inferomedially as the medial malleolus. The distal end of the tibia, when compared with the proximal end, is rotated externally [16–19].

The smooth anterior surface of the distal end of tibia protrudes from the distal surface. It is then separated from the distal surface by a narrow groove, continuing the lateral surface of the shaft. The medial surface of the tibia is smooth and continuous above and below with the medial surfaces of the shaft and malleolus, where it is subcutaneous and visible. The posterior surface of the tibia is intersected near its medial end by a slightly oblique to the vertical groove, extending to the posterior surface of the medial malleolus. The posterior surface of the tibia is smooth and continuous with the posterior surface of the shaft. The lateral surface is the triangular fibular notch, which is bound by ligaments to the fibula. Proximal to the interosseous border, the anterior and posterior edges of the tibia project and converge. Here, a substantial interosseous ligament roughens the floor of the notch proximally. However, the notch remains smooth distally, and is sometimes covered by articular cartilage. Articulating with the talus, the distal surface is wider anteriorly, concave sagittally, and slightly convex transversely. It runs into the malleolar articular surface medially. This articular surface may extend into the groove separating it from the anterior surface of the shaft. Medially or laterally, or both medially or laterally, there are facets that articulate with corresponding talar facets in extreme dorsiflexion [7,10–12,16–18].

The short and thick medial malleolus has a smooth lateral surface with a crescentic facet that articulates with the medial talar surface. It is rough anteriorly and posteriorly, and it continues the groove on the posterior surface of the shaft of the tibia. The distal border points slightly anteriorly, and it is depressed posteriorly. The medial malleolus ends proximal to the lateral malleolus, which is also in a more posterior plane. The posterior groove hosts the tendon of tibialis posterior, which is usually separated from the tendon of flexor digitorum longus by a bone ridge. The capsule of the ankle joint is connected to an anterior groove close to the articular surface. The flexor retinaculum is connected to the groove for the tibialis posterior tendon, on its prominent medial border. Proximal to the distal malleolar border, the deltoid ligament is connected to its apex and depression [7,12,16–18].

The talus, the only tarsal bone with no muscular or tendinous attachments, has seven articulations that connect it to the four other bones. Thus, the stability of the talus and its articulations is provided by the ligamentous attachments and musculotendinous complexes that traverse the talus and attach distally. Several factors act on the passive stability of the ankle joint: the bone stability provided by contact of the trochlea with the tibial plafond; the medial and lateral cartilaginous slightly concave surfaces that articulate with the two malleoli; the ligamentous connections between tibia, fibula, talus, and calcaneus [7,10–12,16–20].

The distal tibiofibular joint is between the rough, medial convex surface on the distal end of the fibula, and the rough concave surface of the fibular notch of the tibia. These are separated distally for about 4 mm by a synovial expansion from the ankle joint, and may be covered by articular cartilage in its lowest part. The joint is generally considered a syndesmosis [16–18].

Ligamentous anatomy of the ankle

Lateral ligaments

The lateral collateral ligamentous complex (from anterior to posterior) is composed of three parts: the anterior talofibular ligament (ATFL), the calcaneofibular ligament (CFL), and the posterior talofibular ligament (PTFL) (Fig. 1).

The ATFL, blending with the anterior capsule of the ankle, courses from the anterior part of the lateral malleolus to the anterior part of the talus. It is the ligament most often involved in inversion ankle sprains [7,10–12,16–18]. In the anatomic position of the foot, the ATFL runs almost horizontally. When the foot is plantarflexed, the ligament is nearly parallel to the long axis of the leg (Fig. 2). In the latter position only, the ligament comes under strain and is vulnerable to injury, particularly when the foot is inverted [21]. ATFL is the weakest of the lateral ankle ligaments, having an ultimate tensile strength of 140 ± 24 N. In biomechanical studies, it has been shown that with incompetence of the lateral ankle ligaments, the resultant anterolateral

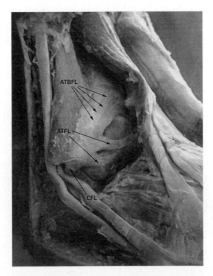

Fig. 1. Lateral ligamentous complex of the ankle (*right*). ATFL, anterior talofibular ligament; CFL, the calcaneofibular ligament; ATBFL, anterior tibiofibular ligament.

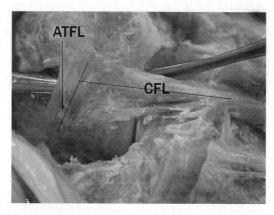

Fig. 2. Angle between the ATFL and the CFL is important for the ankle stability (*left ankle*). ATFL, anterior talofibular ligament; CFL, the calcaneofibular ligament.

rotational instability allows the talus to internally rotate and anteriorly sublux on the tibia [8,22–24].

The CFL is about 2 mm wide, and constitutes the middle portion of the lateral collateral ligamentous complex. Taut between the inferior part of the lateral malleolus to the calcaneus and running in a slightly posterior oblique direction toward the heel, the CFL lies deep to the peroneal tendons, forming a hammock while avoiding these tendons and reaching the calcaneus surface. The angle between the anterior talofibular ligament and the calcaneofibular ligament is important for the ankle stability (Fig. 2).

It is difficult to appreciate the PTFL at ultrasonography because it is partially or at times completely hidden by the lateral malleolus, and courses from the posterior part of the lateral malleolus to the posterior part of the talus [7,10–12,16–18].

Medial ligamentous complex

The deltoid ligament is formed by four or five main ligaments on the medial side. Four are always present: from anterior to posterior, they are the anterior talotibial ligament, the tibionavicular ligament, the calcaneotibial ligament (CTL), and the posterior talotibial ligament (PTTL) (Fig. 3). Sometimes, a calcaneonavicular ligament can be part of the deltoid ligament. The CTL and the PTTL form a superficial layer that runs from the tibia to the sustentaculum tali, and the three others form the deeper layer of the deltoid ligament [7,10–12,16–18].

Inferior tibiofibular joint ligaments

As well as the interosseous membrane, three ligaments, that is, the interosseous tibiofibular ligament, the anterior tibiofibular ligament, and the

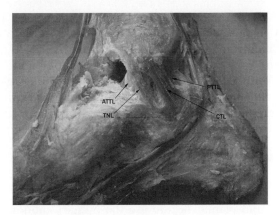

Fig. 3. Medial ligamentous complex of the ankle (*right*). ATTL, anterior talotibial ligament; TNL, the tibionavicular ligament; CTL, calcaneotibial ligament; PTTL, posterior talotibial ligament.

posterior tibiofibular ligament, are present at the joint between the distal tibia and the fibula [7,16–18].

The interosseous tibiofibular ligament, a distal continuation of the interosseous membrane, lies approximately 4 to 5 cm above the level of the ankle joint line (ie, the horizontal part of the joint line between the distal aspect of the tibia and the upper aspect of the trochlea of the talus). It forms a fibrous network that nearly fills the space between the two bones [7,10–12,16–18].

The anterior tibiofibular ligament has three parts, all of which run relatively obliquely in a lateral and distal direction, approximately at 30° to the horizontal (Fig. 4). The parts are separated by a space about 2 mm wide. Both the tibial and the fibular insertions are firmly rooted in the

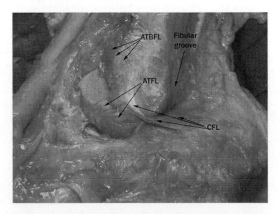

Fig. 4. Anterolateral structures of the ankle (*right*). ATFL, anterior talofibular ligament; CFL, the calcaneofibular ligament; ATBFL, anterior tibiofibular ligament.

cortex. As the tibial insertion is wider than the fibular one, the upper and lower margins of the ligament slightly converge in a lateral and distal direction, giving it a trapezoid shape [7,10–12,16–18].

The posterior tibiofibular ligament and the anterior tibiofibular ligament have similar shapes, although the posterior tibiofibular ligament is fully compact and runs more horizontally. Differentiation of its proximal margin and the interosseous tibiofibular ligament is sometimes challenging, as there is no solution of continuity [7,10–12,16–18].

Functional anatomy and biomechanics

Dorsiflexion and plantar flexion are the primary motions of the ankle, whose axis of rotation is obliquely oriented with regard to all three anatomic planes. The axis extends from anterior, superior, and medial to inferior, posterior, and lateral while passing through the inferior tips of the malleoli. The axis is angled 93° with respect to the long axes of the tibia, and about 11.5° to the joint surface. Rather than a true single instant center of rotation, the ankle has multiple instant centers, which fall very close to a single point within the body of the talus. There may be a shift of the center by a complete arch of ankle rotation anywhere from 4 to 7 mm. Given the oblique orientation of the axis of rotation to the sagittal, coronal, and transverse planes, translations of the talus in the mortise can occur in all three directions [20,25–29].

In vitro studies have shown that the talus rotates easily in the ankle mortise, implying relative movement between the malleoli. The trochlea is wider anteriorly than posteriorly, with an average difference of 4.2 mm. Thus, a lateral shift of the talus within its mortise may occur in plantarflexion of the ankle, while some authors believe that instability exists in dorsiflexion, or that, with intact ligaments, translation occurs only sagittally. The behavior of the ligaments and the roles played by the subtalar joint, the kinematic change of the hindfoot, and the muscles that traverse this area in transmitting forces across the ankle during plantarflexion and dorsiflexion can account for these differences [20].

The normal ankle yields approximately 15° to 20° of active dorsiflexion and between 45° to 55° of active plantar flexion. The maximal dorsiflexion is approximately 10° during the stance phase of normal running and 14° for plantar flexion. Similar to most joints with passive range of motion greater than active ranges, on full weight-bearing ankle passive dorsiflexion is up to 40° [20,30].

External rotation of the talus of 5° to 6° during both active and passive ankle dorsiflexion has been reported [5,20,30]. On plantar flexion, the talus undergoes internal rotation because of its conical and wedge shape. The talus also supinates slightly during plantar flexion [18,20]. Therefore, during dorsiflexion, the talus must pronate. This may be important in tibiofibular ligament injuries associated with dorsiflexion and external rotation [30].

The fibula moves axially, although this movement is not correlated to the degree wedging of the upper talar surface, and there is a change in the axis of rotation of the talus [26]. Another study demonstrated "a slight lateral motion of the fibula at the syndesmosis" was in addition to fibular axial motion [31]. In relation to the tibia, the fibula migrates distally during weight bearing [32]. The fibular movement was attributed to contraction of the flexor muscles of the foot, and it is possible that distal migration of the fibula tightens the intraosseous membrane and deepens the mortise of the ankle joint. Ahl and colleagues [33] showed by a roentgen stereophotogrammetric analysis that in the normal, unloaded ankle, the fibula moves laterally and posteriorly when the ankle moves from plantar flexion into dorsiflexion. In addition, Lofvenberg and colleagues [33] established distal migration of the fibula during adduction of the hindfoot.

In recurrent sprains of the ankle or chronic ankle instability, consideration of some risk factors contribute to planning appropriate management. The risk factors can be evaluated as extrinsic or intrinsic factors [14]. Extrinsic risk factors include some environmental variables such as the level of play, exercise load, amount and standard of training, position played, equipment, playing field conditions, rules, foul play, and so forth. The intrinsic risk factors are based on the individual characteristics of a person. Intrinsic factors include anatomic variations, strength deficits, history of ankle sprain, generalized joint laxity, ankle inversion weakness, limited range of motion, and sex [2]. In addition to intrinsic factors such as diminished muscle strength, postural control, and proprioception and delayed muscle reaction time, the most important ones are biomechanical changes related to anatomic variations [13,34–36].

Anatomic variations underlying recurrent instability have been recently studied. Changes in alignment of the distal tibia, inferior tibiofibular joint pathologies, rotation pathologies of the fibula and their location in the ankle, variations in mortise, variations in the talus morphology, tibiofibular malalignment, cavus foot, and hindfoot malalignment, peroneal muscle weakness, and lateral ankle ligaments constitute some of these variants. Soft tissue problems from structural and traumatic lesions of the ligamentous structures of the ankle such as tibiofibular ligaments, deltoid ligament, and subtalar ligaments are some of the other reasons [37–41].

The stability of the ankle joint depends on the passive stability imparted by ligamentous structures, and on active stability from muscular support. As the talus has no muscular attachment, its stability depends on bony contours and ligamentous integrity. These relationships make the ankle ligaments susceptible to injury [8,22]. The ATFL is vulnerable during plantar flexion, and is thus the most frequently torn ligament following an inversion injury.

A posterior position of the fibula at the ankle mortise could predispose to chronic ankle instability [42]. Scranton and colleagues [42] performed

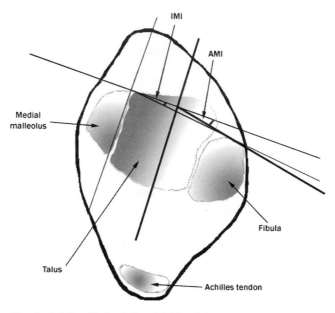

Fig. 5. Axial malleolar index (AMI) and intermallolar index (IMI).

50% of the lateral ankle reconstructions on patients who had a posteriorly positioned fibula. The authors used the "malleolar index" (Fig. 5) to evaluate axial malleolar relationship. They reviewed the CT scans of 100 consecutive patients with a variety of conditions to determine the normal adult variation in the malleolar index. The mean malleolar index was $9.3° \pm 6.5°$. They confirmed that the malleolar index varies from $-12°$ to $+26°$ within a range of $38°$. Berkowitz and Kim [43] studied the relationship between lateral ankle instability and fibular position. In the CT/MRI scans of 65 patients who had lateral ankle stability and underwent stabilization, the malleolar index was $17° \pm 6°$, while this value was $9° \pm 4°$ for the control group. They hypothesized a strong relationship between posterior fibular position and chronic ankle instability requiring surgical reconstruction, and supported the concept of an "open ankle mortise" in patients with a posterior fibula. They suggested that the patients with a more posterior fibula may benefit from early prophylactic bracing and aggressive rehabilitation. Early bracing may protect such patients from recurrent injury, and render the anterior talofibular ligament functionally competent.

A similar study of 61 patients with acute ankle sprain and 101 normal controls showed a statistically poor correlation between the number of sprains and malleolar index [34], with no significant relationship between recurrence of the injury and a higher malleolar index. Thus, static anatomic factors may not contribute to injury until the body is in movement.

In another study on anatomic variations in mortise anatomy, the relationship between the fibula and the medial malleolous was evaluated, and a new method was proposed (Fig. 5). In this study, when the axial malleolar index was measured [22,42], there were significant differences between the control group and patients with recurrent lateral ankle instability. However, when the medial malleolus was considered a reference in the proposed measurement method, there were no significant differences between the two groups. Indeed, it is possible that the position of the medial malleolus is more standard and reproducible [22]. A posteriorly positioned fibula associated with ankle instability may not be a true pathologic entity, but it may instead be the result of measuring from an internally rotated talus [3,22].

The fibula seems to be positioned significantly more anterior in relation to the tibia in subjects with unilateral chronic ankle instability and the more anterior position was a predisposing factor to injury: repetitive bouts of ankle instability caused the fibula to migrate anteriorly [44].

McDermott and colleagues [45] evaluated the MRI of 100 consecutive adult patients for variations in fibular positions, talar length, and anterior talofibular ligament length, predisposing factors of chronic lateral ankle instability. They also obtained MRI of 20 cadavers and dissected them. There was not correlation between malleolar index and talar length or ATFL length. Thus, the fibula appears to play a major role. The fibula descends during stance phase to deepen the mortise. The more posterior the fibula, the greater the vulnerability to ankle sprain and the less the contribution of the lateral malleolus to structural stability of the mortise.

Kanbe and colleagues [46] evaluated the relationship between the shape of tibial plafond and the anterior drawer sign using stress radiographs in patients with severe chronic lateral instability and normal controls. No significant correlation was detected between the anterior drawer sign and talar tilt. However, a significant correlation was found between the anterior tip ratio (ATR) and the anterior drawer sign. Furthermore, the posterior tip ratio, the ankle mortise angle (AMA) and the anterior drawer sign were not correlated. AMA shows the inclination of the lateral tibial plafond, while ATR represents the depth of anterior ankle mortise. The significance of the correlation between the anterior drawer sign and the ATR in chronic lateral instability indicates the importance of the extent of the talus by the anterior tip of the tibia. Sugimoto and colleagues [47] also reported that the varus tilt of the tibial plafond was more often seen in patients with chronic instability of the ankle than in patients with acute ligament sprains.

Van Bergeyk and colleagues [48] investigated hindfoot alignment, another anatomic risk factor in ankle instability. Eleven patients with ankle instability and 12 controls were evaluated by CT: the central calcaneal varus angle was significantly different in the control and study groups. Despite the limited number of patients, the study shows that hindfoot varus is an important predisposing factor in ankle instability.

Barbaix and colleagues [1] considered anatomic variations of the subtalar joint complex to lead to chronic lateral instability of the ankle. They noted that more transverse orientation of the anterior facet of the subtalar joint resulted in greater stability on inversion of the calcaneus.

Svoboda and colleagues [49] investigated the effect of tibial malrotation on tibiotalar joint biomechanics: the pressure applied on the joint on internal and eternal rotations greater than 20° was significantly higher. This suggests a role for tibial torsion, in particular tibiofibular torsion, or more specifically fibular torsion in ankle instability. Tabrizi and colleagues [50] reported limited dorsiflexion to be predisposing for ankle injuries in children. Limited dorsiflexion is observed in patients with low ability of fibula rotation.

The dynamic characteristics of the fibula are not affected only by the ankle or distal tibiofibular joint, but also by the proximal tibiofibular joint [51–54]. If the proximal tibiofibular joint is of the oblique type, the fibula rotates less. Thus, it is a risk factor for injuries of both the knee joint and ankle joint. Given the abnormal dynamic features of the fibula, the triceps surae cannot absorb energy appropriately, and the mechanical loads on the bones and ligaments increase, constituting a predisposing factor for ankle injury [51,53,55].

In basic military trainees, Hurtig and Henderson [56] detected increased prevalence of lower extremity overuse syndrome including ankle injuries with lower hamstring flexibility. Similarly, Bozkurt and colleagues [57] reported that, in patients with short hamstring or hamstring tightness, in addition to lateral knee pain and low back pain associated with the dynamic features of the fibula, ankle problems are observed.

All the variations or changes in the bony or soft tissue anatomy discussed above distort the dynamics of the entire lower extremity, constituting risk factors for ankle injuries. Identification of these factors should allow better planning to prevent ankle injuries, and contribute in planning definitive management in symptomatic instability.

Acknowledgment

We very much appreciate the assistance of Ayhan Comert for his help in anatomic dissections and preparing illustration.

References

[1] Barbaix E, van Roy P, Clarys JP. Variants of anatomical elements contributing to subtalar joint stability: intrinsic risk factors for post-traumatic lateral instability of the ankle. Ergonomics 2000;43:1718–25.

[2] Baumhauer JF, Alosa DM, Renstrom PAFH, et al. A prospective study of ankle injury risk factors. Am J Sports Med 1995;23:564–70.

[3] Berlet GC, Anderson RB. Chronic lateral ankle instability. Foot Ankle Clin 1999;4:713–28.

[4] Bremer SW. Unstable ankle mortise: functional ankle varus. J Foot Ankle Surg 1985;24: 313–7.

[5] Close JR. Some applications of the functional stability of the ankle joint. J Bone Joint Surg Am 1956;38:761–81.

[6] Hertel J. Functional anatomy, pathomechanics, and pathophysiology of lateral ankle instability. J Athl Train 2002;37:364–75.

[7] Hintermann B. Biomechanics of the unstable ankle joint and clinical implications. Med Sci Sports Exerc 1999;31(7 Suppl):S459–69.

[8] Hollis JM, Blasier RD, Flahiff CM. Simulated lateral ankle ligamentous injury: change in ankle stability. Am J Sports Med 1995;23:672–7.

[9] Holmer P, Sondergaard L, Konradsen L, et al. Epidemiology of sprains in the lateral ankle and foot. Foot Ankle Int 1994;15:72–4.

[10] Mann R. Overview of the foot and ankle biomechanics. In: Jahss MH, editor. Disorders of the foot and ankle. Medical and surgical management. 2nd edition. Philadelphia (PA): WB Saunders; 1991.

[11] Myerson M. Current therapy in foot and ankle surgery. St Louis (MO): Mosby Yearbook; 1993.

[12] Safran MR, Benedetti RS, Bartolozzi AR, et al. Lateral ankle sprains: a comprehensive review. Part 1: etiology, pathoanatomy, histopathogenesis, and diagnosis. Med Sci Sports Exerc 1999;31(7 Suppl):S429–37.

[13] Scranton PE. Sprains and soft tissue injuries. In: Pfeffer GB, editor. Chronic ankle pain in athlete. Rosement (IL): AAOS; 2000. p. 3–21.

[14] Willems TM, Witvrouw E, Delbaere K, et al. Intrinsic risk factors for inversion ankle sprains in male subjects. Am J Sports Med 2005;33:415–22.

[15] Brostroem L. Sprained ankles: treatment and prognosis. Acta Chir Scand 1966;132: 537–50.

[16] Williams PL, Bannister LH, Berry MM, et al. editors. Ankle and foot. In: Gray's anatomy. 38th edition. London: Churchill Livingstone; 1999. p. 712–36.

[17] Moore KL, Dalley AFII, Agur AMR. Clinically oriented anatomy. 5th edition. Philadelphia (PA): Lippincot Williams & Wilkins; 2006. p. 702–15.

[18] Sarrafian SK. Anatomy of the foot and ankle. Philadelphia (PA): Lippincott; 1994.

[19] Lundberg A. Kinematics of the ankle and foot: in vitro roentgen stereophotogrammetry. Acta Orthop Scand 1989;60(Suppl 230):1–24.

[20] Simon SR, Alaranta H, An K, et al, editors. Kinesiology. In: Orthopaedic basic science. Boston: American Academy of Orthopaedic Surgeons; 2000. p. 797–800.

[21] Kumai T, Takakura Y, Rufai A, et al. The functional anatomy of the human anterior talofibular ligament in relation to ankle sprains. J Anat 2002;200:457–65.

[22] LeBrun CT, Krause JO. Variations in mortise anatomy. Am J Sports Med 2005;33: 852–5.

[23] McCullough CJ, Burger PD. Rotatory stability o the load bearing ankle. An experimental study. J Bone Joint Surg Br 1980;62:460–4.

[24] Rasmussen O. Stability of the ankle joint: analysis of the function and traumatology of the ankle ligaments. Acta Orthop Scand 1985;(Suppl 211):1–75.

[25] Attarian DE, McCrackin HJ, Devito DP, et al. Biomechanical characterisitics of the human ankle ligament. Foot Ankle 1985;6:54–8.

[26] Barnett CH, Napier JR. The axis of rotation at the ankle joint in man: its influence upon the form of the talus and mobility of the fibula. J Anat 1952;86:1–9.

[27] Lundberg A, Svennson OK, Nemeth G, et al. The axis of the rotation of the ankle joint. J Bone Joint Surg Br 1989;71:94–9.

[28] Rasmussen O, Tovberg-Jensen I. Mobility of the ankle joint. Acta Orthop Scand 1982;53: 155–60.

[29] Sammarco J. Biomechanics of the ankle: surface velocity and instatnt center of rotation in the sagittal plane. Am J Sports Med 1988;16:501–11.

[30] Norcus SA, Floyd RT. The anatomy and mechanisms of syndesmotic ankle sprains. J Athl Train 2001;36(1):68–73.

[31] Scranton PE Jr, McMaster JG, Kelly E. Dynamic fibular function: a new concept. Clin Orthop 1976;118:76–81.

[32] Weinert CR Jr, McMaster JH, Ferguson RJ. Dynamic function of the human fibula. Am J Anat 1973;138(2):145–9.

[33] Ahl T, Dalen N, Lundberg A, et al. Mobility of the ankle mortise. A roentgen stereophoto-grammetric analysis. Acta Orthop Scand 1987;58(4):401–2.

[34] Eren OT, Kucukkaya M, Kabukcuoglu Y, et al. The role of a posteriorly positioned fibula in ankle sprain. Am J Sports Med 2003;31:995–8.

[35] Lentell G, Baas B, Lopez D, et al. The contributions of proprioceptive deficits, muscle function, and anatomic laxity to functional instability of the ankle. J Orthop Sports Phys Ther 1995;21:206–15.

[36] Löfvenberg R, Karrholm J, Sundelin G, et al. Prolonged reaction time in patients with chronic lateral instability of the ankle. Am J Sports Med 1995;23:414–7.

[37] Larsen E, Angermann P. Association of ankle instability and foot deformity. Acta Orthop Scand 1990;61:136–9.

[38] Larsen E, Lund PM. Peroneal muscle function in chronically unstable ankles: a prospective and postoperative electromypgraphic study. Clin Orthop 1991;272:219–26.

[39] Riemann BL. Is there a link between chronic ankle instability and postural instability? J Athl Train 2002;37:386–93.

[40] Rosenbaum D, Becker HP, Sterk J, et al. Functional evaluation of the 10-year outcome after modified Evans repair for chronic ankle instability. Foot Ankle Int 1997;18: 765–71.

[41] Trevino SG, Davis P, Hecht PJ. Management of acute and chronic lateral ligament injuries of the ankle. Orthop Clin North Am 1994;25:1–16.

[42] Scranton PE Jr, McDermott JE, Rogers JV. The relationship between chronic ankle instability and variations in motrise anatomy and impingement spurs. Foot Ankle Int 2000;21:657–64.

[43] Berkowitz MJ, Kim DH. Fibular position in relation to lateral ankle instability. Foot Ankle Int 2004;25:318–21.

[44] Hubbard TJ, Hertel J, Sherbondy P. Fibular position in individuals with self reported chronic ankle instability. J Orthop Sports Phys Ther 2006;36:3–9.

[45] McDermott JE, Scranton PE Jr, Rogers JV. Variations in fibular position, talar length, and anterior talofibular ligament length. Foot Ankle Int 2004;25:625–9.

[46] Kanbe K, Hasegawa A, Nakajima Y, et al. The relationship of the anterior drawer sign to the shape of the tibial plafond in chronic lateral instability of the ankle. Foot Ankle Int 2002;23: 118–22.

[47] Sugimoto K, Samoto N, Takakura Y, et al. Varus tilt of the tibial plafond as a factor in chronic ligament instability. Foot Ankle Int 1997;18:402–5.

[48] Van Bergeyk AB, Younger A, Carson B. CT analysis of hindfoot alignment in chronic lateral ankle instability. Foot Ankle Int 2002;23:37–42.

[49] Svoboda SJ, McHale K, Belkoff SM, et al. The effects of tibial malrotation on the biomechanics of the tibiotalar joint. Foot Ankle Int 2002;23(2):102–6.

[50] Tabrizi P, McIntyre WM, Quesnel MB, et al. Limited dorsiflexion predisposes to injuries of the ankle in children. J Bone Joint Surg Br 2000;82:1103–6.

[51] Bozkurt M, Elhan A, Tekdemir I, et al. An anatomical study of the meniscofibular ligament. Knee Surg Sports Traumatol Arthrosc 2004;12:429–33.

[52] Bozkurt M, Yavuzer G, Tonuk E, et al. Dynamic function of the fibula. Gait analysis evaluation of three different parts of the shank after fibulectomy: proximal, middle and distal. Arch Orthop Trauma Surg 2005;125:713–20.

[53] Bozkurt M, Yilmaz E, Akseki D, et al. The evaluation of the proximal tibiofibular joint for patients with lateral knee pain. Knee 2004;11:307–12.

[54] Bozkurt M, Yilmaz E, Atlihan D, et al. The proximal tibiofibular joint: an anatomic study. Clin Orthop Relat Res 2003;406:136–40.

[55] Jones RB, Ishiwaka SN, Richardson EG, et al. Effects of distal fibular resection on ankle instability. Foot Ankle Int 2001;22:590–3.

[56] Hartig DE, Henderson JM. Increasing hamstring flexibility decreases lower extremity overuse injuries in military basic trainees. Am J Sports Med 1999;27(2):173–6.

[57] Bozkurt M, Can F, Erden Z, et al. The influence of lateral tightness on lateral knee pain. Pain Clin 2004;16:343–8.

ELSEVIER
SAUNDERS

Foot Ankle Clin N Am
11 (2006) 465–474

FOOT AND
ANKLE CLINICS

Management of Recurrent Subluxation of the Peroneal Tendons

Nicholas Antonio Ferran, MBBS, MRCSEd[a],
Nicola Maffulli, MD, PhD, FRCS (Orth)[a],*,
Francesco Oliva, MD[b]

[a]*Department of Trauma and Orthopaedic Surgery, Keele University School of Medicine,
Hartshill, Thornburrow Drive, Stoke-on-Trent, Staffordshire, United Kingdom ST4 7QB*
[b]*University of Rome "Tor Vergata," Faculty of Medicine and Surgery, Department of
Orthopaedics and Traumatology, Viale Oxford 81, 00133 Rome, Italy*

Subluxation of the peroneal tendons is an uncommon sports injury [1], first described in a ballet dancer by Monteggia in 1803 [2]. It is often associated with skiing [1], ice skating, soccer, basketball, rugby, and gymnastics [3]. Acute subluxation usually occurs during forced dorsiflexion of the foot, causing the peroneal muscles to strongly contract [4]. In acute peroneal subluxation, conservative management is associated with a high rate of recurrence, and high-demand individuals should probably be primarily managed surgically [5]. Untreated or misdiagnosed acute injuries predispose patients to recurrent peroneal dislocation [6].

Anatomy

The lateral compartment of the leg contains the peroneal muscles. Peroneus longus originates from the head and upper two-thirds of the peroneal surface of the fibula and from the intermuscular septa. Peroneus brevis originates from the lower two-thirds of the fibula. In the middle third of the fibula, its origin lies in front of that of the peroneus longus, and the two muscles and their tendons maintain this relationship. The broad tendon of peroneus brevis lies immediately posterior to the lateral malleolus. The narrower tendon of peroneus longus lies on that of peroneus brevis. The peroneus brevis tendon passes above the peroneal trochlea of the calcaneus to insert into the tubercle at the base of the fifth metatarsal. The tendon of

---

* Corresponding author.
E-mail address: n.maffulli@keele.ac.uk (N. Maffulli).

1083-7515/06/$ - see front matter © 2006 Elsevier Inc. All rights reserved.
doi:10.1016/j.fcl.2006.06.002   *foot.theclinics.com*

peroneus longus passes below the peroneal trochlea, and passes obliquely to insert into the lateral aspect of the base of the first metatarsal and the medial cuneiform [7]. The peroneal muscles are innervated by the superficial peroneal nerve, and receive their blood supply from the posterior peroneal artery and branches of the medial tarsal artery. Peroneus brevis acts to evert and plantarflex the foot, while peroneus longus everts the foot and assists in plantarflexion of the ankle and first ray.

The retrofibular groove is formed not by the concavity of the fibula itself but by a relatively pronounced ridge of collagenous soft tissue blended with the periosteum that extends along the posterolateral lip of the distal fibula [5]. The shape of the groove is primarily determined by this thick fibrocartilagenous periosteal ridge, and not by the bone itself [4]. Edwards, examining 178 fibulae, noted that a sulcus was present in the bone in 82% of cases, the bone was flat in 11%, and 7% had convex surfaces [8].

The two peroneal tendons are bound to the lateral malleolus by the superior peroneal retinaculum, a band of deep fascia that extends from the posterior aspect of the lateral malleolus to the lateral surface of the calcaneus [7]. The superior peroneal retinaculum is extremely variable in width, thickness, and insertional patterns, with most specimens having insertions on both the calcaneus and the Achilles tendon [9].

The sural nerve, a branch of the tibial nerve, supplies the posterior and lateral skin of the distal third of the leg, proceeding distal to the lateral malleolus along the lateral aspect of the foot and fifth toe [10]. It descends between the heads of gastrocnemius, pierces the deep fascia proximally in the leg, and is joined by a sural communicating branch of the common peroneal nerve. It descends lateral to the Achilles tendon, near the small saphenous vein, to the region between the lateral malleolus and the calcaneus. Its proximity to the peroneal groove needs to be considered when planning surgery, as incisional entrapment can cause painful neuromas and transection results in loss of sensation to the lateral aspect of the foot.

Pathology

The superior peroneal retinaculum is the primary restraint to subluxation of the peroneal tendons in the fibular groove. Eckert and Davis described three grades of acute tears of the superior retinaculum; a fourth grade was later described by Ogden (Fig. 1). In grade 1, the retinaculum is separated from the collagenous lip and lateral malleolus. In grade 2, the collagenous lip is elevated with the retinaculum. In grade 3, a thin sliver of bone, visible on radiographs, is avulsed with the collagenous lip and the retinaculum [5]. In grade 4, the retinaculum is torn away from its posterior attachment on the calcaneus [1]. The superior peroneal retinaculum itself generally remains intact [5]. Clinical determination of injury grade is not possible, except for grade 3 injuries, which can be diagnosed on radiographs.

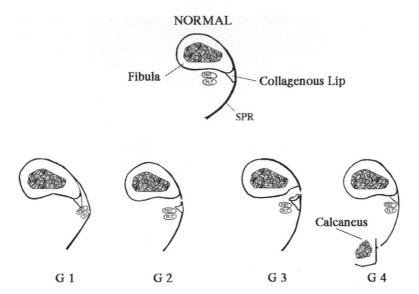

Fig. 1. Diagram of classification of acute tears of the superior peroneal retinaculum (SPR). PBT, peroneus brevis tendon; PLT, peroneus longus tendon.

Peroneal tendon subluxation is commonly associated with longitudinal splits in the peroneus brevis tendon and lateral ankle instability. In the region where the peroneus brevis tendon passes through the fibular groove, the tendon is nearly avascular. Longitudinal splits in the peroneus brevis tendon occur in this region as the tendon subluxes over the sharp collagenous ridge [11]. In cadaveric studies, disruption of the lateral collateral ankle ligaments places considerable strain on the superior peroneal retinaculum. This explains why the two conditions commonly coexist [12].

Clinical features

Patients with recurrent subluxation usually give a history of previous ankle injury often misdiagnosed as a sprain. An unstable ankle that gives way or is associated with a popping or snapping sensation is commonly described. The peroneal tendons may actually be seen subluxing anteriorly on the distal fibula during ambulation (Fig. 2) [13]. Positioning the patient prone with the knees flexed at 90°, with active dorsiflexion and plantar flexion and eversion against resistance, may demonstrate the dynamic instability of the tendons [14].

Although radiographs are helpful in diagnosing grade 3 injuries to the superior peroneal retinaculum [15], diagnosis is primarily made on clinical grounds, and imaging modalities are not widely used. Dynamic high-resolution ultrasound can be effective in demonstrating subluxation and associated tendon splits [16,17]. CT may be helpful in assessing the retrofibular

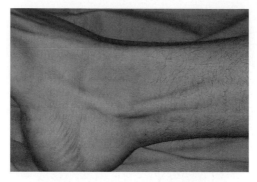

Fig. 2. Subluxation of peroneal tendons.

groove before, and postoperatively in, groove-deepening procedures [18]. Static MRI is useful in grading superior peroneal retinaculum injuries, identifying splits in the peroneal tendons, diagnosing abnormality in the lateral collateral ankle ligament complex, and demonstrating morphologic abnormalities of the fibular groove (flat, convex, or irregular) [19].

Management

Although conservative management may be attempted in acute dislocations, recurrent dislocations should be managed surgically [20–27]. Various surgical techniques have been described. However, no randomized studies have been conducted to determine which method of treatment is superior, and the available literature is limited to case reports and small case series.

There are five categories of surgical repair: (1) anatomic reattachment of the retinaculum, (2) reinforcement of the superior peroneal retinaculum with local tissue transfers, (3) rerouting the tendons behind the calcaneofibular ligament, (4) bone block procedures, and (5) groove deepening procedures [3].

The aim of anatomic reattachment of the retinaculum is restoration of the primary restraint to the peroneal tendons. Reattachment with sutures brought through drill holes in the distal fibula has been described [5,28–32]. As an alternative, Beck [22] brought the retinaculum through a slit created in the distal fibula and fixed this with a screw, and treated nine patients without complication. Eighteen of 21 patients treated with the "Singapore operation" at 9 years had excellent results. However, three patients experienced postoperative pain and neuromas; no recurrence was noted [33]. Karlsson and colleagues reported 13 patients with good to excellent results that were able to return to full activity, and two patients whose activity were limited by pain; no recurrence were noted at follow-up. They did, however, employ groove deepening in conjunction with reattachment if the posterior surface of the fibula was flat or convex [32].

Several authors have described procedures to augment or reinforce an attenuated retinaculum with tissue transfers consisting of either tendon or periosteal flaps. Ellis Jones [34] first described restraining the peroneal tendons with a strip of Achilles tendon anchored through a drill hole in the fibula. No recurrences were noted in a long-term follow-up of 15 patients who underwent the Ellis-Jones repair [35]. Thomas and colleagues [6] described a modification to this procedure that allowed the use of a smaller strip of Achilles tendon, reducing the risk of weakening the tendon. Use of the tendon of peroneus brevis [36–38], plantaris [39,40], and peroneus quartus [41] have been described for the same purpose. Zoellner and Clancy [42] and Gould [43] used periosteal flaps to restrain the peroneal tendons in a deepened peroneal grove with satisfactory results. In patients treated with a periosteal flap from the retrofibular grove on its own or incorporated with groove deepening, no postoperative complications were noted [44].

The use of the calcaneofibular ligament (CFL) as an alternative restraint has been considered. Platzgummer [45] described dividing the CFL and transposing the tendons behind it; 13 patients operated with this technique showed good or excellent results, with no evidence of recurrence or instability [46]. Sarmiento and Wolf later divided the peroneal tendons and reattached them after rerouting them behind the CFL [47]; 11 patients showed no evidence of recurrence or instability at follow-up, although 2 patients suffered sural nerve injury [48]. Both methods may potentially weaken these structures. To preserve CFL integrity, a bone block of the ligamentous insertion on the fibula [49] or the calcaneus [25] is mobilized, the tendons are transposed, and the bone block is reattached with a screw. Pozo and Jackson [49] reported no complications and return to full level of activity in a case report. Poll and Duijfjes [25] reported 10 patients with no recurrence or instability.

Bone block procedures were developed to deepen the retrofibular groove using a bone graft as a physical restraint to the peroneal tendons. In 1920, Kelly [50] described a bone block procedure using screw fixation for the sliding veneer graft but later designed a wedge-shaped graft that avoided the use of screws near the ankle joint. DuVries and Watson-Jones [51] modified Kelly's technique. Watson-Jones [52] used an osteoperiosteal flap anchored by a soft tissue pedicle and secured it posteriorly with sutures. DuVries anchored a posteriorly displaced wedge with a screw. Other authors reported on patients with chronic subluxation operated with a modified Kelly technique with no recurrence [21,23,53]. Larsen and colleagues [24] and Lowry and colleagues [54] reported on the DuVries technique. Larsen and colleagues reported many complications including intraarticular screw, fracture of the malleolus, fracture of the graft, nonunion, redislocation and pain associated with the screw, but Lowry and colleagues noted no complications in a case report. In 1989, Micheli and colleagues [55] treated 12 patients with an inferiorly displaced fibula bone graft fixed with screws; one suffered a traumatic fracture of the graft, and two required exploration for pain; no recurrences were noted. Tendon adhesion to the fresh bone wound, fractures of bone grafts, and the need for metalwork are major disadvantages of bone block procedures [22].

The depth of the retrofibular sulcus was previously thought to play an important role in the restraint of the peroneal tendons, thus leading to the development of procedures to deepen the sulcus when it was found to be flat or convex. Zoellner and Clancy [48] elevated an osteoperiosteal flap posteriorly on the distal fibula and removed cancellous bone with a gauge. The flap was then reduced into the deepened sulcus, and the tendons replaced into this. Their nine patients had excellent results with no recurrence or instability. Hutchinson and Gustafson described a similar method in combination with superior peroneal retinaculum (SPR) reattachment. Of 20 patients, 3 had poor results with resubluxation, and one of these developed reflex sympathetic dystrophy [56]. Gould [49] reported a single patient in whom groove deepening was incorporated with restraint of the peroneal tendons by reflection of elevated osteoperiosteal flaps. Mendicino and colleagues [57] employed intramedullary drilling and cortical impaction to achieve groove deepening. The need for groove deepening has been questioned. Anatomic studies demonstrate the incidence of a flat or convex sulcus as high as 18% [8], 28% [25], and 30% [58]. The low incidence of peroneal tendon subluxation would suggest that the bony sulcus is not a predisposing factor to subluxation [8]. Histologic studies demonstrating that the peroneal groove is defined by the fibrocartilagenous periosteal cushion and not the bony sulcus add weight to this argument [4].

We prefer an anatomic approach to the management of peroneal tendon subluxation and opt for SPR reattachment (Maffulli et al, accepted for publication, *Am J Sports Med*). Under general or spinal anesthetic, the patient is placed supine with a sandbag under the buttock of the operative side. A tourniquet is applied to the thigh, the leg exsanguinated, and the cuff inflated to 250 mmHg.

A 5-cm longitudinal incision is made along the course of the peroneal tendons, staying well anterior to the sural nerve. The peroneal tendon sheath is incised longitudinally. The SPR is normally thin and deficient, especially anteriorly. The peroneal tendons are identified, inspected, and protected. If a tear of the peroneal tendons is found, this is repaired with fine absorbable sutures. The lateral aspect of the lateral malleolus is exposed, and the "pouch" formed between the bony surface of the lateral malleolus and the SPR becomes visible.

The bony surface of the lateral malleolus is roughened up, and three or four anchors are inserted along the posterior border of the fibula (Fig. 3). The SPR is reconstructed in a "vest-over-pants" fashion, making sure that the pouch between the bony surface of the lateral malleolus and the SPR is obliterated (Fig. 4). The ankle is kept in eversion and slight dorsiflexion so that the peroneal tendons are in the "worst possible position." The strength of the repair is tested moving the ankle through a range of motion.

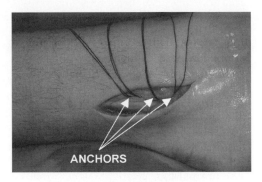

Fig. 3. Anchor and sutures in situ.

The wound is closed in layers with 2/0 vicryl (Ethicon, Edinburgh, UK) for the subcutaneous fat, subcuticular undyed 3/0 vicryl (Ethicon, Edinburgh, UK), and steristrips (3M, Loughborough, UK). Dressing swabs, dressing, and crepe bandage are applied. A below-knee walking synthetic cast is applied with the ankle in neutral and slight eversion. Weight bearing is allowed from the day after the operation, and the plaster is removed four weeks after the procedure, when rehabilitation is started. Gradual return to activities is allowed over the course of 3 to 4 months from the procedure. Patients are allowed to return to their sport on the fifth postoperative month.

In the period 1996 to 2001, we operated on 14 patients (all men; mean age, 25.3 ± 6.3 years; range, 18–37 years). All had sustained a traumatic unilateral peroneal tendon subluxation: six playing soccer, three playing basketball, three playing rugby, and two having fallen off a motor bike. In five patients, the peroneal tendon subluxation had not been diagnosed at the time of injury, and the patients were told that they had sustained an inversion sprain of the ankle. The mean time between injury and surgery was 10.1 ± 2.5 months (range, 7–19 months).

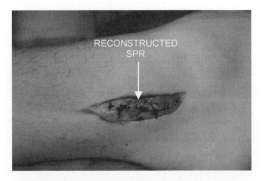

Fig. 4. Superior peroneal retinaculum is reconstructed.

Patients were reviewed in a special clinic during 4 consecutive weeks at a mean of 38 ± 3 months (range, 22–47 months) after the operation. Two patients did not attend, as they lived too far away: both were asymptomatic, and were interviewed by telephone.

No patient experienced a further episode of peroneal tendon subluxation at final review, and all had returned to their normal activities of daily living and their sports activities. In particular, of the six soccer players, two were still engaged in their sport but less frequently. The three basketball players had returned fully to their sport, and one of the three rugby players had become a coach. The two patients who had fallen off a motor bike were able to conduct an otherwise normal life.

Summary

Recurrent peroneal tendon subluxation when an acute injury is misdiagnosed or not adequately managed. The primary pathology is failure of the SPR, the principal restraint to the peroneal tendons.

Several surgical techniques have been described. Determining the most effective technique from the small case series and reports in the literature is impossible. If an anatomic approach to treating the pathology is used, reattachment of the SPR, as we have described, seems a most appropriate technique. Rarely, the retinaculum in recurrent cases may not be robust enough to withstand repair, and a different approach to the problem may be required. In the future, there may be an emerging role for minimally invasive SPR repair with the use of endoscopic techniques.

References

[1] Oden RR. Tendon injuries about the ankle resulting from skiing. Clin Orthop 1987;216: 63–9.
[2] Monteggia GB. Instituzini chirurgiche, part III. Milan (Italy): Pirotta E Maspero; 1803. p. 336–41.
[3] Mizel MS. Orthopedic knowledge update. Foot and ankle 2. Rosemont (IL): American Academy of Orthopedic Surgeons; 1998.
[4] Kumai T, Benjamin M. The histological structure of the malleolar groove of the fibula in man: its direct bearing on the displacement of the peroneal tendons and their surgical repair. J Anat 2003;203:257–62.
[5] Eckert WR, Davis EA Jr. Acute rupture of the peroneal retinaculum. J Bone Joint Surg Am 1976;58(5):670–2.
[6] Thomas JL, Sheridan L, Graviet S. A modification of the Ellis Jones procedure for chronic peroneal subluxation. J Foot Surg 1992;31(5):454–8.
[7] Sinnatamby CS. Last's anatomy regional and applied. 10th edition. Edinburgh: Churchill Livingstone; 1999. p. 1–518.
[8] Edwards ME. The relation of the peroneal tendons to the fibula, calcaneus, and cuboideum. Am J Anat 1928;42:213–53.
[9] Davis WH, Sobel M, Deland J, et al. The superior peroneal retinaculum: an anatomic study. Foot Ankle Int 1994;15(5):271–5.

[10] Williams PL. Gray's anatomy. 38th edition. London: Churchill Livingstone; 1995.
[11] Petersen W, Bobka T, Stein V, et al. Blood supply of the peroneal tendons: injection and immunohistochemical studies of cadaver tendons. Acta Orthop Scand 2000;71(2):168–74.
[12] Geppert MJ, Sobel M, Bohne WH. Lateral ankle instability as a cause of superior peroneal retinacular laxity: an anatomic and biomechanical study of cadaveric feet. Foot Ankle 1993; 14(6):330–4.
[13] Niemi WJ, Savidakis J Jr, DeJesus JM. Peroneal subluxation: a comprehensive review of the literature with case presentations. J Foot Ankle Surg 1997;36(2):141–5.
[14] Safran MR, O'Malley D Jr, Fu FH. Peroneal tendon subluxation in athletes: new exam technique, case reports, and review. Med Sci Sports Exerc 1999;31(7 Suppl):S487–92.
[15] Church CC. Radiographic diagnosis of acute peroneal tendon dislocation. AJR Am J Roentgenol 1977;129(6):1065–8.
[16] Neustadter J, Raikin SM, Nazarian LN. Dynamic sonographic evaluation of peroneal tendon subluxation. AJR Am J Roentgenol 2004;183(4):985–8.
[17] Magnano GM, Occhi M, Di Stadio M, Toma' P, Derchi LE. High-resolution US of nontraumatic recurrent dislocation of the peroneal tendons: a case report. Pediatr Radiol 1998;28(6):476–7.
[18] Szczukowski M Jr, St Pierre RK, Fleming LL, et al. Computerized tomography in the evaluation of peroneal tendon dislocation. A report of two cases. Am J Sports Med 1983;11(6): 444–7.
[19] Rosenberg ZS, Bencardino J, Astion D, et al. MRI features of chronic injuries of the superior peroneal retinaculum. AJR Am J Roentgenol 2003;181(6):1551–7.
[20] Brage ME, Hansen ST Jr. Traumatic subluxation/dislocation of the peroneal tendons. Foot Ankle 1992;13(7):423–31.
[21] McLennan JG. Treatment of acute and chronic luxations of the peroneal tendons. Am J Sports Med 1980;8(6):432–6.
[22] Beck E. Operative treatment of recurrent dislocation of the peroneal tendons. Arch Orthop Trauma Surg 1981;98(4):247–50.
[23] Wobbes T. Dislocation of the peroneal tendons. Arch Chir Neerl 1975;27(3):209–15.
[24] Larsen E, Flink-Olsen M, Seerup K. Surgery for recurrent dislocation of the peroneal tendons. Acta Orthop Scand 1984;55(5):554–5.
[25] Poll RG, Duijfjes F. The treatment of recurrent dislocation of the peroneal tendons. J Bone Joint Surg Br 1984;66(1):98–100.
[26] Tan V, Lin SS, Okereke E. Superior peroneal retinaculoplasty: a surgical technique for peroneal subluxation. Clin Orthop 2003;410:320–5.
[27] Kollias SL, Ferkel RD. Fibular grooving for recurrent peroneal tendon subluxation. Am J Sports Med 1997;25(3):329–35.
[28] Alm A, Lamke LO, Liljedahl SO. Surgical treatment of dislocation of the peroneal tendons. Injury 1975;7(1):14–9.
[29] Das De S, Balasubramaniam P. A repair operation for recurrent dislocation of peroneal tendons. J Bone Joint Surg Br 1985;67(4):585–7.
[30] Smith TF, Vitto GR. Subluxing peroneal tendons. An anatomic approach. Clin Podiatr Med Surg 1991;8(3):555–77.
[31] Mason RB, Henderson JP. Traumatic peroneal tendon instability. Am J Sports Med 1996; 24(5):652–8.
[32] Karlsson J, Eriksson BI, Sward L. Recurrent dislocation of the peroneal tendons. Scand J Med Sci Sports 1996;6(4):242–6.
[33] Hui JH, Das De S, Balasubramaniam P. The Singapore operation for recurrent dislocation of peroneal tendons: long-term results. J Bone Joint Surg Br 1998;80(2):325–7.
[34] Jones E. Operative treatment of chronic dislocation of the peroneal tendons. Bone Joint Surg 1932;14:574–6.
[35] Escalas F, Figueras JM, Merino JA. Dislocation of the peroneal tendons. Long-term results of surgical treatment. J Bone Joint Surg Am 1980;62(3):451–3.

[36] Arrowsmith SR, Fleming LL, Allman FL. Traumatic dislocations of the peroneal tendons. Am J Sports Med 1983;11(3):142–6.

[37] Gurevitz SL. Surgical correction of subluxing peroneal tendons with a case report. J Am Podiatry Assoc 1979;69(6):357–63.

[38] Stein RE. Reconstruction of the superior peroneal retinaculum using a portion of the peroneus brevis tendon. A case report. J Bone Joint Surg Am 1987;69(2):298–9.

[39] Miller JW. Dislocation of peroneal tendons—a new operative procedure. A case report. Am J Orthop 1967;9(7):136–7.

[40] Hansen BH. Reconstruction of the peroneal retinaculum using the plantaris tendon: a case report. Scand J Med Sci Sports 1996;6(6):355–8.

[41] Mick CA, Lynch F. Reconstruction of the peroneal retinaculum using the peroneus quartus. A case report. J Bone Joint Surg Am 1987;69(2):296–7.

[42] Zoellner G, Clancy W Jr. Recurrent dislocation of the peroneal tendon. J Bone Joint Surg Am 1979;61(2):292–4.

[43] Gould N. Technique tips: footings. Repair of dislocating peroneal tendons. Foot Ankle 1986;6(4):208–13.

[44] Lin S, Tan V, Okereke E. Subluxating peroneal tendon: repair of superior peroneal retinaculum using a retrofibular periosteal flap. Tech Foot Ankle Surg 2003;2(4):262–7.

[45] Platzgummer H. Uber ein einfaches Verfahren zur operativen Behandlung der habituellen Peronaeussehnenluxation. Arch Orthop Unfallchir 1967;61:144–50.

[46] Sarmiento A, Wolf M. Subluxation of peroneal tendons. Case treated by rerouting tendons under calcaneofibular ligament. J Bone Joint Surg Am 1975;57(1):115–6.

[47] Steinbock G, Pinsger M. Treatment of peroneal tendon dislocation by transposition under the calcaneofibular ligament. Foot Ankle Int 1994;15(3):107–11.

[48] Martens MA, Noyez JF, Mulier JC. Recurrent dislocation of the peroneal tendons. Results of rerouting the tendons under the calcaneofibular ligament. Am J Sports Med 1986;14(2): 148–50.

[49] Pozo JL, Jackson AM. A rerouting operation for dislocation of peroneal tendons: operative technique and case report. Foot Ankle 1984;5(1):42–4.

[50] Kelly RE. An operation for the chronic dislocation of the peroneal tendons. Br J Surg 1920;7: 502.

[51] Watson-Jones R. Fractures and joint injuries. 4th edition. Baltimore (MD): Williams & Wilkins; 1956.

[52] DuVries HL. Surgery of the Foot. 4th edition. St. Louis (MO): C.V. Mosby Co.; 1978.

[53] Marti R. Dislocation of the peroneal tendons. Am J Sports Med 1977;5(1):19–22.

[54] Lowy A, Kruman N, Kanat IO. Subluxing peroneal tendons. Treatment with the use of an autogenous sliding bone graft. J Am Podiatr Med Assoc 1985;75(5):249–53.

[55] Micheli LJ, Waters PM, Sanders DP. Sliding fibular graft repair for chronic dislocation of the peroneal tendons. Am J Sports Med 1989;17(1):68–71.

[56] Hutchinson BL, Gustafson LS. Chronic peroneal tendon subluxation. New surgical technique and retrospective analysis. J Am Podiatr Med Assoc 1994;84(10):511–7.

[57] Mendicino RW, Orsini RC, Whitman SE, et al. Fibular groove deepening for recurrent peroneal subluxation. J Foot Ankle Surg 2001;40(4):252–63.

[58] Mabit C, Salanne PH, Blanchard F, et al. The retromalleolar groove of the fibula: a radio-anatomical study. Foot Ankle Surg 1999;5:179–86.

ELSEVIER
SAUNDERS

Foot Ankle Clin N Am
11 (2006) 475–496

FOOT AND
ANKLE CLINICS

Diagnosis and Imaging of Ankle Instability

James F. Griffith, FRCR[a,*],
Jason Brockwell, FRCSEd (Orth)[b]

[a]*Department of Diagnostic Radiology & Organ Imaging, Chinese University of Hong Kong,
Shatin, Hong Kong*
[b]*Sports Physicians, 8/F, AON China Building, 29 Queen's Road Central, Hong Kong*

Ankle injuries are common, with a crude incidence of about 60 per 10,000 in the general population [1], and constituting 11% of all soccer injuries [2]. Most settle with no, or simple, conservative measures, but the huge volume makes them an important clinical problem. In addition, some progress to chronicity, and it is difficult to predict which. Patients may have a variety of problems after an injury, including instability, impingement, and articular cartilage damage. We present a simple practical approach to ankle instability diagnosis and imaging.

History

Presenting complaint

Patients presenting with frank instability—the ankle giving way—are relatively uncommon. They often present following an acute injury, or complaining of pain. Further questioning may reveal a previous history of instability or a "weak ankle".

Pain

In a recent injury, pain is often felt over the injured structures, typically the anterior talofibular ligament (ATFL), at times associated with pain at the base of the fifth metatarsal and Lisfranc joint, less commonly over the deltoid ligament or the syndesmosis. The location of pain (and tenderness)

---

* Corresponding author.
E-mail address: griffith@cuhk.edu.hk (J.F. Griffith).

1083-7515/06/$ - see front matter © 2006 Elsevier Inc. All rights reserved.
doi:10.1016/j.fcl.2006.07.001

is diagnostic. Chronic pain is usually anterior and superficial, and worse on dorsiflexion, implying anterior impingement. The pain can be posterior and deep, and worse on plantarflexion, implying posterior impingement, or nonspecific and deep, often worse on impact, for instance descending stairs, implying articular cartilage injury. Medial gutter pain may be associated with medial instability [3].

Instability

Patients may volunteer, or admit on questioning, a history of giving way of the ankle, often with minor provocation, such as uneven pavement, or may report that the ankle feels "weak." Often this symptom follows the first episode of injury, which is usually noted to be more major than subsequent injuries.

Injury

It is useful to know the mechanism of any injury. Inversion injuries are most common, and typically involve the ATFL, and less commonly the calcaneofibular ligament (CFL) with an associated posteromedial talar dome injury. Eversion injuries are less common, and typically involve the deltoid ligament, with an anterolateral talar dome injury. Rotation injuries are more common in certain sports, for instance ice hockey [4], and increasingly common in rugby due to tackle rule changes, and involve the syndesmosis. Higher energy injuries, such as landing badly from a jump, are more commonly associated with articular cartilage damage than lower energy injuries such as a stumble.

Previous injury

Prior injuries are common. Typically there is a history of a normal ankle suffering a significant sprain, often with difficulty weightbearing lasting several weeks, followed by chronic or recurrent symptoms. Often there has been little rehabilitation.

Swelling

The location of any swelling is helpful: in acute injuries, it is often over the injured structures. In both acute and chronic circumstances there may be diffuse swelling along the joint line.

Management

The management of both present and any previous complaints should be noted. If there has been inadequate rehabilitation, a trial of physiotherapy supervised strength and proprioception exercises may be appropriate. If there were symptoms despite adequate rehabilitation, one would consider surgery.

Other side

It is important to know whether the contralateral ankle has been injured, and whether it is symptomatic, as it is helpful to have a "normal" side for comparison at examination.

General history

A thorough general history, even in "simple" cases, such as an acute ankle sprain, will reduce the chance of being caught out.

Occupation

Apart from professional sportsmen, certain occupational groups have increased demand or may be at increased risk from an ankle giving way, for example, steeplejacks and scaffolders.

General health

Obviously, generalized diseases such as dementia influence management of ankle problems; equally, some generalized diseases have specific effects on the ankle, such as impaired proprioception in diabetes or peroneal weakness in Charcot-Marie-Tooth disease [5], polio [5,6], or other forms of paralysis [7].

Past medical history

A history of patellar or shoulder dislocations may point toward generalized ligamentous laxity. A history of tuberculosis should make one even more suspicious of this great mimic [8].

Family history

A family history of Charcot-Marie-Tooth or collagen diseases is a give away, but a family history of "ankle problems" may point to the above diagnoses.

Sport

An individual's sports participation is usually vital to management of ankle problems, as in many cases symptoms only occur during sport.

Drug history

There are no drugs that definitely specifically affect the ankle, but a full drug history should be noted, especially supplements and alternative medicines. The "supplement" glucosamine is used in osteoarthritis, but takes 3 to 4 weeks to produce pain relief, and the dose is not universally agreed, though 1500 mg/d is recommended [9]. If it is being used, one should note dose and duration of use before drawing conclusions about its effectiveness [9]. Some alternative or traditional medicines contain powerful synthetic steroids, which can obviously greatly affect the progress of an ankle problem, as well as masking the symptoms and signs of infection and predisposing to avascular necrosis of bone. Quinolone antibiotics are known to cause Achilles tendon problems [10], and one study has shown lesions in the articular cartilage of rats' ankles [11].

Examination

General

One cannot examine the ankle in isolation: it is necessary to examine the whole person, but particularly the overall gait, and examine in detail the whole of both legs and both feet. Naturally, examination begins with overall impression: general appearance, dress, and appropriateness of manner. Test generalized ligamentous laxity using the Carter-Wilkinson score [12], although it may not correlate with ankle laxity [13]. Generalized ligamentous laxity may predispose to ankle injuries [14]. Systems examination is guided by history, and unless the history is suggestive, systems examination is not performed.

Gait, footwear, braces, and orthotics

Note the gait in shoes with any orthotics or braces. Inspect the footwear for its appropriateness, age, and pattern of wear. Check the condition and fit of any orthotics or braces. Assess the stability (see below) of the ankle in and out of any brace. Note the gait in bare feet. Check the ability to walk both on tiptoes and on the heels, and to squat keeping the heels on the ground: with limited ankle dorsiflexion the heels will rise. With a varus heel, perform a Coleman block test to identify a fixed plantarflexed first ray as a contributing cause [15]; this may require a first metatarsal osteotomy in addition to a calcaneal osteotomy to correct the deformity and allow successful lateral ligament stabilization [15].

Appearance

Inspect the legs, ankles and feet for shape, deformity, swelling, bruising, callosities and the condition of the skin and nails, noting carefully any side-to-side differences. Look for wasting of the peroneal compartments consistent with Charcot-Marie-Tooth. Inspection from above will give a broad impression of whether the shape of the foot is normal, cavovarus, predisposing to lateral instability [15], or planovalgus, associated with both medial [16] and lateral instability [17]. Inspection from behind will demonstrate whether the Achilles tendon is in line with the tibia or curving in valgus or varus. One may see "too many toes" in planovalgus feet. With the patient seated or standing and a little weight through the leg, find the talar neutral position by grasping the anterior process of the talus between thumb and index and forefingers, and move the subtalar joint from eversion to inversion and back until one can "feel" that the talus is neutral. In pronated feet, this will often lift the first metatarsal head off the floor, and cavus feet are often demonstrated to be high arched but pronated. With the patient prone or kneeling on a chair and with the foot hanging free, find the talar neutral while viewing from behind to assess forefoot angle relative to the hindfoot.

Tenderness

Palpate for tenderness of defined anatomic structures. In an acute injury, the Ottawa Ankle Rules recommend no radiographs unless the individual cannot bear weight and has tenderness of the posterior aspect of one of the malleoli or the base of the fifth metatarsal [18–20]. Palpate the ATFL, CFL, and deltoid ligaments for tenderness. Palpate the syndesmosis noting how far proximally any tenderness of the anterior border of the fibula extends: in syndesmosis sprains, each centimeter of tenderness represents about an extra day off competitive sport from a baseline of 5 days off [21]. Anterior joint line tenderness is associated with impingement and articular cartilage damage [22].

Swelling

Swelling is usual over the injured structures. A joint effusion will be visible as diffuse swelling across the anterior joint line and confirmed by fluctuation. Pressure is transmitted from the posterior joint to the anterior aspect of the joint if the posterior joint is compressed by squeezing Kager's fat pad between fingers placed anterior to and on either side of the Achilles tendon.

Range of motion

Note the ranges of motion of the ankle with the knees flexed and extended, and the range of motion subtalar and midfoot joints.

Tendon function

Each tendon crossing the ankle joint must be tested by resisting its action and feeling for tightening of the tendon or contraction of its muscle. It is not easy to distinguish a single peroneal tendon rupture, which is probably why they are rarely reported [23] (Fig.1), but other tendon ruptures are usually clinically apparent. In particular, one should note peroneal strength. Peroneal subluxation or dislocation may be painless [24].

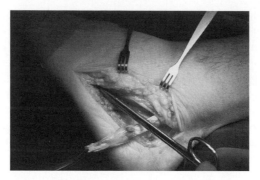

Fig. 1. Traumatic peroneus longus rupture from inversion injury.

Ankle ligaments

The anterior drawer and inversion tests are used to assess the lateral ankle ligaments. The hindfoot is grasped in neutral with one hand, and the distal tibia is grasped with the other. The hindfoot is drawn anteriorly, and the amount of movement and character of the endpoint estimated, and compared with the other side [25]. There is disagreement over how much, if any, axial load should be applied. Axial loading will reduce the amount of translation, probably reducing sensitivity [26–28]. The inversion test is performed by inverting the hindfoot relative to the tibia [29]. In neutral, the ATFL is the major resistor of anterior talar displacement and the CFL is the major resistor of inversion. In maximal plantar flexion, resistance to inversion is shared between the CFL and the ATFL [30]. These tests are reasonably accurate for diagnosing ligament injury, although not very accurate at quantifying the severity of the injury, and may be subject to false negatives [31]. The normal range of motion may be reduced by muscle spasm secondary to pain, and some authors recommend performing these tests under local or general anesthesia [31,32], although this is not generally accepted. Women have more physiologic laxity than men [33]. To quantify motion, various researchers have developed instrumented devices and demonstrated reasonable accuracy compared with stress radiographs [34,35], although no device is widely used. However, given the present lack of clinical usefulness of this information, the devices are likely to remain research tools for the time being [36].

The deltoid ligament is similarly assessed by manual eversion, lateral translation, and drawer tests [37], although medial instability may be overshadowed by concurrent lateral instability, and is probably best diagnosed by arthroscopy [38].

The syndesmosis is assessed by pain provoking tests: external rotation of the talus in the mortise; the "squeeze test"—squeezing the tibia and fibula together; and attempted weightbearing in plantarflexion—which is limited by pain and weakness in a syndesmosis injury [21,39]. It is difficult to elicit abnormal mobility in syndesmotic injuries [40].

It is difficult to differentiate subtalar instability from lateral ankle instability [41].

Neurologic and vascular

Ankle instability may be secondary to neurologic deficit, especially in the cavovarus foot, and one should check for adequate blood supply.

Special investigations

Footprint

If available, a pressure mat, which displays the pressure of the footprints and center of gravity, can aid understanding. The shape and peak pressures of the footprint provide information about the foot. The center of gravity may be deviated to stabilize the foot—compensatory pronation with the center of gravity medialised will help to prevent inversion in lateral ankle instability [17,42], although a similar appearance may be present in medial instability [16].

A 1 or 2-m long pressure mat allows for a more natural walk (or run), as it is very difficult to place a footstep cleanly on a small pressure mat.

Video running assessment

A video analyzed running assessment adds information. Simple video analysis software (eg, Dartfish, Swinger, or Silicon Coach) allows the tester to stop motion and analyze angles, for instance, heel varus or valgus (Fig. 2).

EMGs and reaction times

EMG and other special tests to measure muscle reaction times are presently used as research tools, and are unlikely to come into routine clinical practice in the near future [43,44], although simpler force mat and pressure plate devices for quantifying control of balance are easy to use for assessment and rehabilitation and may become popular [43], and may be used in combination with other modalities of assessment [45].

Imaging

Imaging of ankle instability primarily involves assessment of the ankle ligaments but also of the ankle capsules, bones, and tendons.

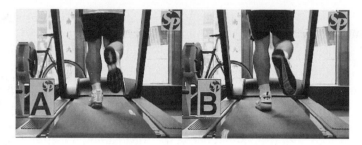

Fig. 2. Video running assessment with (A) normal and (B) motion control shoes.

Radiography

In low- to moderate-energy ankle injuries, such as those associated with athletic activity, the prevalence of fractures around the ankle joint is not high, varying from about 3% to 8% [46]. If a fracture is clinically suspected, radiographs will usually be obtained following initial clinical assessment. Standard radiographs of the ankle for initial assessment include anteroposterior, lateral, and mortise views (Fig. 3). For the mortise view, the patient's leg is internally rotated (by about 20° in males and 15° in females) so that the lateral and medial malleoli are parallel to the tabletop. This view provides a true anteroposterior projection of the ankle mortise and the talar dome. The anteroposterior and mortise views are complementary in fracture detection, and all three views should be obtained for initial assessment. The Ottawa ankle rules [18], or one of their modifications [47], can reduce requests for ankle radiographs by almost half, reducing costs and waiting time. These decision rules have good interobserver agreement among trained clinicians (kappa coefficient 0.8) and a very high negative predictive value (of close to 1.0). This indicates that the likelihood of a fracture being overlooked is low (estimated at around 0.6%) if these rules are properly applied [47]. In addition, the overlooked fractures tend to be clinically irrelevant [47]. The Ottawa ankle rules have only been validated in adults, and have not been specifically tested in children.

Although radiographs are very accurate at revealing fractures around the ankle, radiographically occult fractures occasionally occur. The best indicator of an occult fracture is a large ankle effusion [48]. Ankle effusions are best seen on the lateral radiograph as a homogenous soft tissue-like density displacing the fat plane located anterior to the ankle joint (Fig. 4). A joint effusion resulting in fat plane displacement of >13 mm has a positive predictive value of 82% for occult fracture. The presence of an ankle effusion of >13 mm is a reasonable threshold to consider additional imaging of the ankle by either 45° oblique radiography or computed tomography. However, most radiographically occult fractures around the ankle joint are not displaced, and will not contribute to ankle instability.

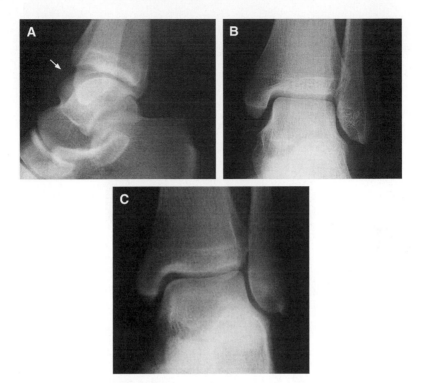

Fig. 3. (*A*) Lateral radiograph of the ankle. Notice normal fat-like density just anterior to ankle joint (*arrow*). (*B*) Frontal (anteroposterior projection). Note the degree to which the fibula overlays the tibia. (*C*) Mortise view. The ankle has been internally rotated providing a clear projection of the ankle joint mortise.

In the acute stage, clinical examination, particularly if performed at about 5 days after injury, has high diagnostic accuracy for ligament tear. When performed correctly, clinical examination depicts the presence of ligament tear with a sensitivity of 96% and a specificity of 84% [49]. Clinical examination is less reliable at distinguishing the severity of a tear, that is, whether the ligament is partially or completely torn. Because the majority of ankle ligament injuries will settle satisfactorily with conservative management, initial imaging is usually confined to radiographic assessment in those patients in whom a fracture is clinically suspected. Either clinical examination alone, or clinical examination followed by radiography, will, in most instances, be sufficient to guide management. More specialized investigations are currently not warranted in the acute setting, as there is no reliable evidence that they will significantly alter patient care.

A minority of patients continue to have pain, limitation of movement, and mechanical or functional instability many months after injury, when they would normally be expected to be almost symptom free. It is in this minority that further imaging is usually indicated. Chronic symptoms may

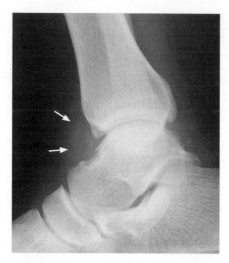

Fig. 4. Lateral radiograph showing a large joint effusion as a homogenous soft tissue density anterior to the ankle joint (*arrows*). Note that capsular thickening in the absence of a large effusion may produce an identical appearance.

stem from a variety of causes, such as ligament injury leading to mechanical instability, osseous or soft tissue impingement leading to impingement, synovitis, osteochondral injury, or para-articular tendinous injury. There is no reliable means of predicting which patients with moderate to severe acute ankle injury will proceed to develop chronic symptoms. Although such a prediction would be extremely useful and may allow better tailored management, there is no evidence that any imaging investigation can reliably select which patients with ligament injury will settle and which will go on to develop chronic sequelae.

Imaging investigations for chronic ankle instability focus on demonstrating the integrity of the ankle ligaments. A variety of imaging investigations are available, with the general trend being a move from radiographic-based examinations to cross-sectional imaging examinations.

Peroneal tenography and ankle arthrography

Peroneal tenography involves injection of contrast medium into the peroneal tendon sheaths under fluoroscopic guidance. The test is designed to show communication between the peroneal tendon sheaths and the ankle joint. This communication is normally absent. The calcaneofibular ligament passes immediately deep to the peroneal tendons. If the calcaneofibular ligament tears, the medial wall of the peroneal tendon sheaths and the ankle capsule usually also tear, and a communication develops between the two compartments (Fig. 5). A positive result is very specific for calcaneofibular ligament injury. The sensitivity and specificity of peroneal tenography for

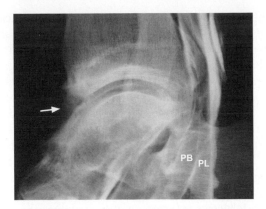

Fig. 5. Peroneal tenography. Contrast medium outlines the peroneus longus (PL) and brevis (PB) tendons. Note how these two tendons share a common tendon sheath behind the lateral malleolus and have separate tendon sheaths distally. The contrast has leaked from the tendon sheaths into the ankle joint (*arrow*).

calcaneofibular ligament tear are 82% and 96%, respectively [50]. In supination injuries of the ankle, the anterior talofibular ligament is the first to tear followed by the calcaneofibular ligament. Isolated calcaneofibular ligament tears are uncommon. The assumption is that if the calcaneofibular ligament is torn, the anterior talofibular ligament is also torn.

Ankle arthrography can be used instead of peroneal tenography. Ankle arthrography involves injection of contrast medium into the ankle joint under fluoroscopic control. Arthrography tends to have a lower sensitivity for calcaneofibular ligament tears than peroneal tenography because contrast medium will take the path of least resistance and may preferentially leak out into the pericapsular tissues rather than into the peroneal tendon sheaths. The sensitivity and specificity of ankle arthrography for calcaneofibular ligament tear is 65% and 46% [50]. Both peroneal tenography and ankle arthrography must be performed soon after injury, ideally within 24 hours, and certainly within 1 week. These tests are of little or no value in chronic ankle instability, because most communicating defects will have sealed.

Stress radiography

Stress radiography (or stress fluoroscopy) is the only imaging investigation to directly demonstrate increased laxity at the ankle. The main limitation of stress radiography is the lack of universally accepted criteria for talar tilt and anterior talar translation [51,52]. Wide ranges of values for normal and injured ankles have been published [52]. Differences in the reported values may originate from physiologic variability, technique variability (instrumentation, method of loading, force, duration of loading, use of anesthesia) and measurement variability (criteria used, intrinsic measurement error).

Stress radiography should only be undertaken when clinical assessment is compatible with instability and when any added information provided will influence treatment. Stress can be applied manually or with a commercially available jig. The main value of using a jig is that the test can be standardized with an applied pressure of up to 150 N. Inversion stress, if applied in plantar flexion, evaluates the anterior talofibular ligament. Applied in neutral dorsiflexion, it assesses both the anterior talofibular and calcaneofibular ligaments. Again, reported values for normal and abnormal vary considerably [52]. Nevertheless, for neutral dorsiflexion, talar tilt of the injured side greater than 15° (Fig. 6a) or a side-to side difference of greater than 10° is commonly recognized as predictive of anterior talofibular and calcaneofibular ligament disruption.

Anterior talar displacement stress mainly evaluates the anterior talofibular ligament. It is measured as the shortest distance from the posterior lip of the tibia to the talar dome, and it may be more predictive than talar tilt. Reported normal and abnormal measurements vary considerably though a pre- and poststress difference of 10 mm and a side-to-side difference of 5 mm is considered pathologic (Fig. 6b). The appropriateness of stress radiography in determining the presence, severity, and cause of ankle instability as well as clinical outcome is questionable, because much of the information provided can be obtained with experienced clinical examination [52,53].

Ultrasonography

Ultrasound is an efficient, dynamic, and noninvasive means of evaluating the ankle ligaments and tendons [54] (Fig. 7). Dedicated equipment with high-frequency transducers and good examination technique are necessary to fully evaluate these structures. The ligaments appear hyperechoic when

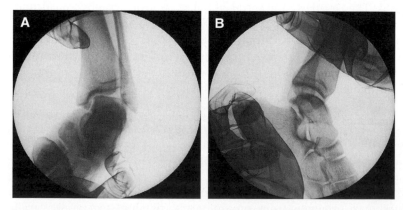

Fig. 6. Stress fluoroscopy. (*A*) Inversion stress in plantar flexion showing a talar tilt of more than 15° indicative of complete anterior talofibular ligament tear. (*B*) Anterior talar displacement showing increased anterior talar displacement indicative of complete anterior talofibular ligament tear.

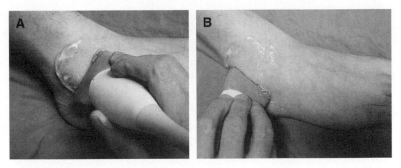

Fig. 7. Transducer position used to demonstrate the (*A*) anterior talofibular ligament and (*B*) the calcaneofibular ligament.

the fibers are parallel to the ultrasound beam (Fig. 8). The ligaments are best visualized when they are stretched by putting the foot in slight plantar flexion for the anterior talofibular ligament and in slight dorsiflexion for the calcaneofibular ligament [55]. The deep component of the medial collateral ligament (deltoid ligament) is best seen by dorsiflexing and slightly everting

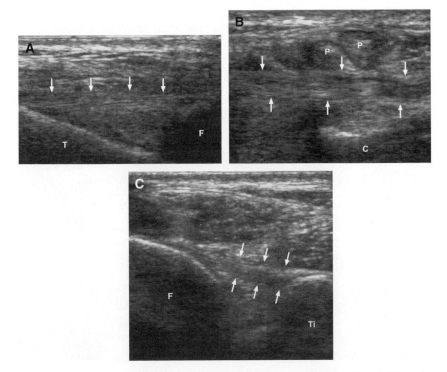

Fig. 8. Ultrasound. (*A*) Oblique transverse image showing a normal anterior talofibular ligament (*arrows*), (*B*) oblique longitudinal image showing a normal calcaneofibular ligament (*arrows*) deep to the peroneal tendons (P), and (*C*) transverse image showing a normal posterior tibiofibular ligament (*arrows*). F, fibula; T, talus; C, calcaneum; Ti, tibia.

the foot [55]. The anterior talofibular and calcaneofibular ligaments are normally about 2 mm wide, while the deltoid ligament is fan shaped.

Ligament tears may be apparent at the insertional areas or centrally within the mid-third of the ligament. Acute ligament injury is seen as ligament swelling, ligament discontinuity, hypoechogenicity (representing fluid or edema) paralleling or transversing the ligament [54], or nonvisualization of the ligament (Fig. 9). In experienced hands, the accuracy of ultrasonography for acute anterior talofibular ligament tears is about 95%; for the calcaneofibular ligament, the accuracy of ultrasonography 90%, and for anterior tibiofibular ligament tears the accuracy is 85% [54].

A healed ligament is usually thickened, although it may occasionally be attenuated. If the ligament does not heal, it either reabsorbs fully, in which case no ligament is visible, or the ligament may retract as a fibrotic mass attached to one of the insertional areas.

MRI

MRI can reliably and consistently demonstrate all of the normal ankle ligaments (Fig. 10). MRI may be performed with the foot in a neural or slightly flexed position. The flexed position helps align the anterior talofibular and calcaneofibular ligaments into true axial or coronal plane so that they can be seen in their entirety on a single image. The flexed position, however, has the disadvantage of being more difficult to maintain, especially if the ankle is painful, and the chance of motion artifact is increased. The

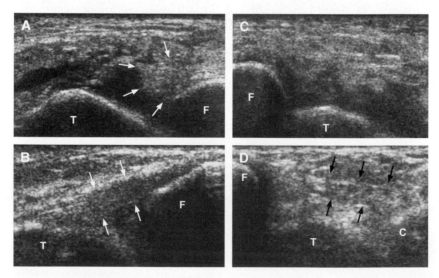

Fig. 9. Ultrasound showing (*A*) complete tear (discontinuity) of anterior talofibular ligament (*arrows*) with (*B*) normal side (*arrows*) for comparison. (*C*) Compete tear (nonvisualization) (*arrows*) of calcaneofibular ligament with (*D*) normal side (*arrows*) for comparison. F, fibula; T, talus; C, calcaneum.

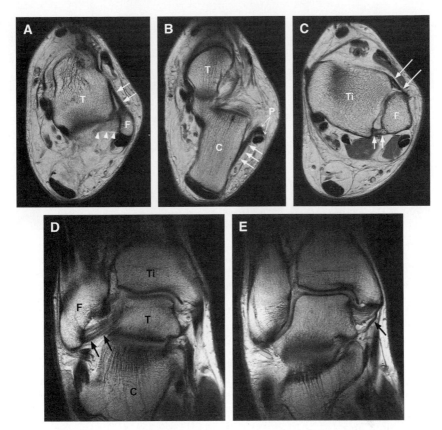

Fig. 10. Magnetic resonance imaging. Intermediate-weighted axial images of the ankle showing (*A*) a normal anterior talofibular ligament (*arrows*) and posterior talofibular ligament (*arrowheads*), (*B*) a normal calcaneofibular ligament (*arrows*) running deep to the peroneal tendons (P), and (*C*) normal anterior tibiofibular (*long arrows*) and posterior tibiofibular (*short arrows*). Intermediate-weighted coronal MR images of the ankle showing (*D*) a normal posterior talofibular ligament (*arrows*) and (*E*) a normal deltoid ligament (*arrow*). F, fibula; T, talus; C, calcaneum; Ti, tibia.

neutral position will provide adequate visualization in most cases. Use of a superficial coil can also improve ligament visibility. The cardinal MRI signs of ligament injury are ligament swelling, discontinuity, a lax or wavy ligament, or nonvisualization (Fig. 11). MRI is also very sensitive at demonstrating the co-occurrence and nature of other injuries such as chondral injury, bone bruising, radiographically occult fractures, sinus tarsus injury, paraarticular tendon tears, or degeneration, and the many causes of impingement syndrome. The main limitations of MRI are cost, time, availability, and motion artifact. MRI-based studies have provided useful confirmatory evidence that the injury spectrum sustained in distal tibiofibular syndesmotic injury is very different to that of inversion ankle injuries,

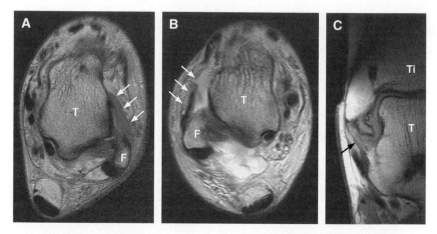

Fig. 11. Magnetic resonance imaging. Intermediate-weighted axial image of the ankle showing (*A*) a severe sprain of anterior talofibular ligament with a swollen though continuous ligament (*arrows*), (*B*) a complete tear (discontinuity) of the anterior talofibular ligament (*arrows*) near the talar insertion, and (*C*) a coronal image showing an old injury of the deltoid ligament (*arrow*). Note how the deltoid ligament has lost its normal wavy appearance. There is a large osteophytic spur protruding from the medial malleolus into the deltoid ligament. F, fibula; T, talus; C, calcaneum; Ti, tibia.

due to the different mechanisms involved. MRI-based studies of acute ankle injury have not shown any specific features that can reliably predict patients that will progress to chronic sequelae following acute ligament injury.

Syndesmotic injury

Injury to the distal tibiofibular syndesmosis ligaments is also known as "high ankle sprain." The ligaments supporting this joint are the anterior or posterior tibiofibular ligaments and the interosseous ligament. The completely torn distal tibiofibular joint diastasis will result in lateral translation of the talus, decreased tibiotalar contact area, and increased tibiotalar contact pressure with predisposition to arthrosis. Injury to the distal tibiofibular syndesmosis can occur in isolation or in combination with ankle fracture. When severe diastasis has occurred, the injury is usually readily apparent on frontal or mortise radiography. Lesser degrees of diastasis may not be readily apparent on radiography. In this situation, measurements made on a standard frontal radiograph are used to help diagnose syndesmotic injury. The accuracy of these measurements has recently been questioned [56,57], as repeat measurements are not reliable, and measurements vary considerably with ankle position. Therefore, one should not rely on radiographic measurements to diagnose syndesmotic injury [56]. Syndesmosis injury will be either apparent on radiography without the need for measurement, or, if clinically suspected in the absence of an unequivocal radiographic abnormality, additional investigation, with MRI, ultrasound, or arthroscopy, should be performed. If one wants assurance of the normality or otherwise of the ankle radiograph, a comparative anteroposterior view of the contralateral normal ankle is more useful than radiographic measurement of the injured side [56,58].

The useful radiographic landmarks that can be reliably demonstrated on an anteroposterior projection of the ankle are (a) the medial clear space (ie, widest distance between the medial border of the talus and the lateral border of the medial malleolus, (b) superior clear space (ie, distance between superior point of medial talus and the tibial plafond), (c) anterior tibial tubercle, and (d) medial border of fibula [56] (Fig. 12). Two radiographic observations are useful. First, a medial clear space greater than the superior clear space on a nonweightbearing radiograph suggests deltoid ligament disruption. Second, absence of overlap between the anterior tibial tubercle and the medial border of the fibula (ie, absence of tibiofibular overlap) suggests syndesmosis diastasis, particularly if this is present on the affected side and not on the contralateral side (because bilateral nontraumatic absence of tibiofibular overlap has been noted) [56].

Positive radiographic evaluation only occurs if there is widening (or diastasis) of the distal tibiofibular syndesmosis. Less severe degrees of syndesmotic ligament tear may occur with little or no diastasis. In such instances, radiography will be negative. When compared with more sensitive investigations such as MRI or arthroscopy, radiography fares poorly in depicting syndesmotic injury. Compared with MRI in 70 patients with ankle fracture, very little correlation was found between radiographic measurement and

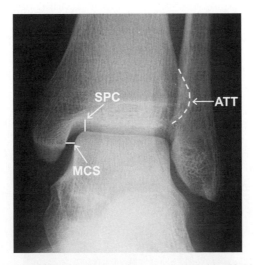

Fig. 12. Anteroposterior radiograph of the ankle showing the identifiable and reliable landmarks for diagnosing syndesmosis diastasis. The medial clear space (MCS) should be less then the superior clear space (SPC). The anterior tibial tubercle (ATT) should overlay the fibula.

syndesmotic injury [57]. The only useful radiographic measure was the medial clear space. This measure correlated well with deltoid ligament injury
and became wider with increasing severity of deltoid ligament injury [57].
Overall, while radiographs will reveal frank syndesmotic diastasis, they
should not be relied upon to detect lesser degrees of syndesmotic injury.

MRI is very sensitive and specific in the diagnosis of syndesmotic ligament injury [59,60]. The criteria for syndesmotic ligament disruption on
MRI are (a) ligament discontinuity, (b) a wavy or lax ligament, and (c) nonvisualization of the ligament (Fig. 13). Using these criteria with arthroscopy
as the "gold standard," the sensitivity and specificity of MRI for ligament
disruption were 100%/93% and 100%/94% for an anterior and posterior
tibiofibular ligament injury, respectively. The third definable syndesmotic
ligament is the intraosseous ligament. This ligament, which is contiguous
with the interosseous membrane, is the shortest and one of the strongest
tibiofibular connections. The intraosseous ligament can also be depicted
on MRI, although no studies have specifically evaluated its accuracy in
depiction of intraosseous ligament disruption.

MR-based studies have provided useful confirmatory evidence that
the injury spectrum in distal tibiofibular syndesmotic injury is very different to that of inversion ankle injuries. Syndesmotic injury occurs as
a result of an eversion–supination injury. As such, anterior tibiofibular
and calcaneofibular ligament injury does not tend to accompany syndesmotic injury, while deltoid ligament injury commonly accompanies this
injury. The accuracy of ultrasound in syndesmotic injury has not been
specifically tested.

In summary, imaging assesses mechanical and not functional instability.
This is achieved directly by stress radiography and indirectly by peroneal tenography, ultrasound, and MRI. Lately, through the application of more

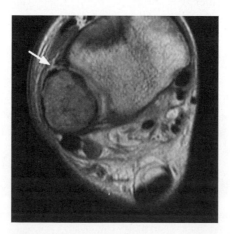

Fig. 13. Intermediate-weighted axial MR image of the ankle showing a tear of the anterior tibiofibular ligament (*arrow*).

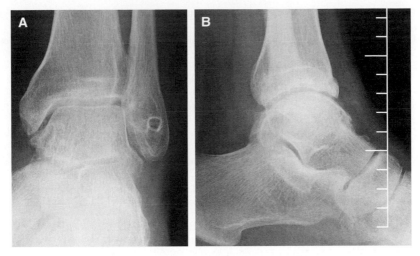

Fig. 14. Radiograph shows (*A*) instability controlled by ligament reconstruction, and (*B*) anterior impingement persists from neglected osteophytes.

sensitive investigative techniques (such as ultrasound, MRI, and arthroscopy), the limitations of radiographic-based techniques (stress radiography, and peroneal tenography) in the assessment of ligament disruption have been highlighted. The current trend is to move from radiographic-based examinations to cross-sectional examinations in the evaluation of ankle instability. Although MRI, and, to a slightly lesser extent, ultrasound, are very accurate in the assessment of acute ankle injury, their routine application in acute ankle injury offers no distinct advantage over clinical assessment, in that the injuries demonstrated have generally little bearing on treatment or outcome prediction. MRI allows a global assessment of ankle injuries, and is likely to be increasingly used as the principal imaging modality in ankle instability.

Summary

Ankle instability is a major cause of symptoms following an ankle sprain. With a thorough history and examination, appropriate additional investigations, including cross-sectional imaging, and thoughtful interpretation of the information, one should rarely be caught out by misdiagnosis, multiple diagnoses (Fig. 14), or unusual underlying causes.

References

[1] Bridgman SA, Clement D, Downing A, et al. Population based epidemiology of ankle sprains attending accident and emergency units in the West Midlands of England, and a survey of UK practice for severe ankle sprains. Emerg Med J 2003;20(6):508–10.
[2] Ekstrand J, Tropp H. The incidence of ankle sprains in soccer. Foot Ankle 1990;11(1):41–4.

[3] Boss AP, Hintermann B. Anatomical study of the medial ankle ligament complex. Foot Ankle Int 2002;23(6):547–53.

[4] Wright RW, Barile RJ, Surprenant DA, et al. Ankle syndesmosis sprains in national hockey league players. Am J Sports Med 2004;32(8):1941–5.

[5] Burns J, Redmond A, Ouvrier R, et al. Quantification of muscle strength and imbalance in neurogenic pes cavus, compared to health controls, using hand-held dynamometry. Foot Ankle Int 2005;26(7):540–4.

[6] Mukherjee A, Varma SK, Natarajan K. Ankle joint instability in poliomyelitis. Indian J Pediatr 1972;39(289):37–8.

[7] Anderson RL, Hills HM Jr, Abplanalp AA. Lateral instability of the ankle in paralytic cases. South Med J 1955;48(7):718–24.

[8] Guttler A, Hammerschmidt S, Wirtz H, et al. Unexpected cause of a tarsal destruction in a diabetic patient. Dtsch Med Wochenschr 2004;129(22):1243–5.

[9] Reginster JY, Deroisy R, Rovati LC, et al. Long-term effects of glucosamine sulphate on osteoarthritis progression: a randomised, placebo-controlled clinical trial. Lancet 2001; 357(9252):251–6.

[10] Waterston SW, Maffulli N, Ewen SW. Subcutaneous rupture of the Achilles tendon: basic science and some aspects of clinical practice. Br J Sports Med 1997;31(4):285–98.

[11] Kashida Y, Kato M. Toxic effects of quinolone antibacterial agents on the musculoskeletal system in juvenile rats. Toxicol Pathol 1997;25(6):635–43.

[12] Carter C, Wilkinson J. Persistent joint laxity and congenital dislocation of the hip. J Bone Joint Surg Br 1964;46:40–5.

[13] Pearsall AW, Kovaleski JE, Heitman RJ, et al. The relationships between instrumented measurements of ankle and knee ligamentous laxity and generalized joint laxity. J Sports Med Phys Fitness 2006;46(1):104–10.

[14] Stewart DRB. Does generalised ligamentous laxity increase seasonal incidence of injuries in male first division club rugby players? Br J Sports Med 2004;38(4):457–60.

[15] Fortin PT, Guettler J, Manoli A 2nd. Idiopathic cavovarus and lateral ankle instability: recognition and treatment implications relating to ankle arthritis. Foot Ankle Int 2002;23(11): 1031–7.

[16] Hintermann B. Medial ankle instability. Foot Ankle Clin 2003;8(4):723–38.

[17] Becker H, Rosenbaum D, Claes L. Measurement of plantar pressure distribution during gait for diagnosis of functional lateral ankle instability. Clin Biomech (Bristol, Avon) 1997;12(3): S19.

[18] Stiell IG, Greenberg GH, McKnight RD, et al. Decision rules for the use of radiography in acute ankle injuries. Refinement and prospective validation. JAMA 1993;269(9):1127–32.

[19] Stiell IG, Greenberg GH, McKnight RD, et al. A study to develop clinical decision rules for the use of radiography in acute ankle injuries. Ann Emerg Med 1992;21(4):384–90.

[20] Stiell IG, McKnight RD, Greenberg GH, et al. Implementation of the Ottawa ankle rules. JAMA 1994;271(11):827–32.

[21] Nussbaum ED, Hosea TM, Sieler SD, et al. Prospective evaluation of syndesmotic ankle sprains without diastasis. Am J Sports Med 2001;29(1):31–5.

[22] van Dijk CN, Bossuyt PM, Marti RK. Medial ankle pain after lateral ligament rupture. J Bone Joint Surg Br 1996;78(4):562–7.

[23] Konradsen L, Sommer H. Ankle instability caused by peroneal tendon rupture. A case report. Acta Orthop Scand 1989;60(6):723–4.

[24] Sobel M, Warren RF, Brourman S. Lateral ankle instability associated with dislocation of the peroneal tendons treated by the Chrisman-Snook procedure. A case report and literature review. Am J Sports Med 1990;18(5):539–43.

[25] Frost HM, Hanson CA. Technique for testing the drawer sign in the ankle. Clin Orthop Relat Res 1977;123:49–51.

[26] Liu W, Maitland ME, Nigg BM. The effect of axial load on the in vivo anterior drawer test of the ankle joint complex. Foot Ankle Int 2000;21(5):420–6.

[27] Ray RG, Christensen JC, Gusman DN. Critical evaluation of anterior drawer measurement methods in the ankle. Clin Orthop Relat Res 1997;334:215–24.

[28] Tohyama H, Yasuda K, Ohkoshi Y, et al. Anterior drawer test for acute anterior talofibular ligament injuries of the ankle. How much load should be applied during the test? Am J Sports Med 2003;31(2):226–32.

[29] Kahan R. Talar tilt following ankle injury. J Am Podiatry Assoc 1959;49(1):20–1.

[30] Bahr R, Pena F, Shine J, et al. Mechanics of the anterior drawer and talar tilt tests. A cadaveric study of lateral ligament injuries of the ankle. Acta Orthop Scand 1997;68(5):435–41.

[31] McCaskie AW, Gale DW, Finlay D, et al. Chronic ankle instability: the value of talar tilt under general anaesthesia. Br J Sports Med 1995;29(2):103–4.

[32] Becker HP, Komischke A, Danz B, et al. Stress diagnostics of the sprained ankle: evaluation of the anterior drawer test with and without anesthesia. Foot Ankle 1993;14(8):459–64.

[33] Wilkerson RD, Mason MA. Differences in men's and women's mean ankle ligamentous laxity. Iowa Orthop J 2000;20:46–8.

[34] Hubbard TJ, Kaminski TW, Vander Griend RA, et al. Quantitative assessment of mechanical laxity in the functionally unstable ankle. Med Sci Sports Exerc 2004;36(5):760–6.

[35] Spahn G. The ankle meter: an instrument for evaluation of anterior talar drawer in ankle sprain. Knee Surg Sports Traumatol Arthrosc 2004;12(4):338–42.

[36] Frost SC, Amendola A. Is stress radiography necessary in the diagnosis of acute or chronic ankle instability? Clin J Sport Med 1999;9(1):40–5.

[37] Quiles M, Requena F, Gomez L, et al. Functional anatomy of the medial collateral ligament of the ankle joint. Foot Ankle 1983;4(2):73–82.

[38] Hintermann B, Valderrabano V, Boss A, et al. Medial ankle instability: an exploratory, prospective study of fifty-two cases. Am J Sports Med 2004;32(1):183–90.

[39] Guise ER. Rotational ligamentous injuries to the ankle in football. Am J Sports Med 1976; 4(1):1–6.

[40] Beumer A, van Hemert WL, Swierstra BA, et al. A biomechanical evaluation of clinical stress tests for syndesmotic ankle instability. Foot Ankle Int 2003;24(4):358–63.

[41] Karlsson J, Eriksson BI, Renstrom PA. Subtalar ankle instability. A review. Sports Med 1997;24(5):337–46.

[42] Nawata K, Nishihara S, Hayashi I, et al. Plantar pressure distribution during gait in athletes with functional instability of the ankle joint: preliminary report. J Orthop Sci 2005;10(3): 298–301.

[43] Munn J, Beard DJ, Refshauge KM, et al. Eccentric muscle strength in functional ankle instability. Med Sci Sports Exerc 2003;35(2):245–50.

[44] Konradsen L, Ravn JB. Prolonged peroneal reaction time in ankle instability. Int J Sports Med 1991;12(3):290–2.

[45] Testerman C, Vander Griend R. Evaluation of ankle instability using the Biodex Stability System. Foot Ankle Int 1999;20(5):317–21.

[46] Garrick JG, Requa RK. The epidemiology of foot and ankle injuries in sports. Clin Sports Med 1988;7(1):29–36.

[47] Springer BA, Arciero RA, Tenuta JJ, et al. A prospective study of modified Ottawa ankle rules in a military population. Am J Sports Med 2000;28(6):864–8.

[48] Clark TW, Janzen DL, Ho K, et al. Detection of radiographically occult ankle fractures following acute trauma: positive predictive value of an ankle effusion. AJR Am J Roentgenol 1995;164(5):1185–9.

[49] van Dijk CN, Lim LS, Bossuyt PM, et al. Physical examination is sufficient for the diagnosis of sprained ankles. J Bone Joint Surg Br 1996;78(6):958–62.

[50] Bleichrodt RP, Kingma LM, Binnendijk B, et al. Injuries of the lateral ankle ligaments: classification with tenography and arthrography. Radiology 1989;173(2):347–9.

[51] Beynnon BD, Webb G, Huber BM, et al. Radiographic measurement of anterior talar translation in the ankle: determination of the most reliable method. Clin Biomech (Bristol, Avon) 2005;20(3):301–6.

[52] Senall JA, Kile TA. Stress radiography. Foot Ankle Clin 2000;5(1):165–84.
[53] Freeman MA. Instability of the foot after injuries to the lateral ligament of the ankle. J Bone Joint Surg Br 1965;47(4):669–77.
[54] Peetrons P, Creteur V, Bacq C. Sonography of ankle ligaments. J Clin Ultrasound 2004; 32(9):491–9.
[55] Campbell DG, Menz A, Isaacs J. Dynamic ankle ultrasonography. A new imaging technique for acute ankle ligament injuries. Am J Sports Med 1994;22(6):855–8.
[56] Beumer A, van Hemert WL, Niesing R, et al. Radiographic measurement of the distal tibio-fibular syndesmosis has limited use. Clin Orthop Relat Res 2004;423:227–34.
[57] Nielson JH, Gardner MJ, Peterson MG, et al. Radiographic measurements do not predict syndesmotic injury in ankle fractures: an MRI study. Clin Orthop Relat Res 2005;436: 216–21.
[58] Pneumaticos SG, Noble PC, Chatziioannou SN, et al. The effects of rotation on radiographic evaluation of the tibiofibular syndesmosis. Foot Ankle Int 2002;23(2):107–11.
[59] Muhle C, Frank LR, Rand T, et al. Tibiofibular syndesmosis: high-resolution MRI using a local gradient coil. J Comput Assist Tomogr 1998;22(6):938–44.
[60] Oae K, Takao M, Naito K, et al. Injury of the tibiofibular syndesmosis: value of MR imaging for diagnosis. Radiology 2003;227(1):155–61.

ELSEVIER
SAUNDERS

Foot Ankle Clin N Am
11 (2006) 497–507

FOOT AND
ANKLE CLINICS

Acute Lateral Ankle Sprains in Track and Field Athletes: An Expanded Classification

Nikolaos Malliaropoulos, MD, MScSpMed, PhD[a],
Emmanuel Papacostas, MD[a], Agapi Papalada, PT[a],
Nicola Maffulli, MD, MS, PhD, FRCS (Orth)[b],*

[a]*National Track & Field Centre, Sports Injury Clinic,
Sports Medicine Clinic of S.E.G.A.S., Thessaloniki, Greece*
[b]*Department of Trauma and Orthopaedic Surgery, Keele University School of Medicine,
Thornburrow Drive, Hartshill, Stoke on Trent ST4 7QB Staffs, United Kingdom*

There has been a recent increase in participation in sport at all levels [1]. Injuries to the lateral ankle ligaments constitute 15% to 45% of all sports-related injuries [2,3], while the crude incidence rate of ankle sprains attending the emergency departments has risen from 60.9 [4] to 70 [5] per 10,000 residents. Underestimating the frequency and the impact of acute ankle ligament injuries leads to poor diagnosis, unsuitable management, and long-term complications. Many physicians rely on their own, at times limited, experience to manage high level athletes. They may therefore inaccurately assess the injury, and over- or underestimate the time needed for full return to sport.

Earlier studies indicate that 85% of ankle sprains involve forced inversion and plantar flexion [6]. Eighty percent of lateral ankle sprain injuries most commonly involve the anterior talofibular ligament (ATFL). In 20%, more violent inversion force damages the calcaneofibular ligament (CFL) as well [4,7].

In our setting, we plan the initial management of ankle sprain according to pain, ability to bear weight, range of motion (ROM), edema (EDE), and stress radiographs. In addition, we routinely measure active ROM, and quantify the presence of EDE by the figure-of-eight method.

We had the clinical impression that the grading of ankle sprains in athletes could be enriched by further subgrouping. Therefore, we felt that

---

* Corresponding author.
E-mail address: n.maffulli@keele.ac.uk (N. Maffulli).

1083-7515/06/$ - see front matter © 2006 Elsevier Inc. All rights reserved.
doi:10.1016/j.fcl.2006.05.004   *foot.theclinics.com*

distinction should be made in athletes with a grade III ankle sprain taking into consideration the results of stress radiographs, the active ROM at presentation, and the total rehabilitation time.

In our own center, over a period of 10 years (Malliaropoulos, Papacostas, Papalada, unpublished data, 2004), 25.4% (309 of 1215) of all sports injuries were ankle injuries without fracture. Acute lateral ligament injuries were 22.4% (272 of 1215). In the present study, 208 track and field athletes, originally diagnosed as suffering from acute lateral ankle injuries, were classified according to severity by using the above criteria. We report the results of a longitudinal observational study on ankle sprains in athletes.

Patients and methods

All procedures reported in the present study were approved by our Institutional Ethics Review Board, and all athletes gave their written informed consent to participate in the study. All patients were examined and assessed by a fellowship trained sports physician.

In the period December 1996 to December 2002, we examined 1215 injured track and field athletes. Of these, 309 (25.43%) were referred because of an ankle sprain, and 272 had injuries of their lateral ligamentous complex. All the patients underwent a thorough clinical examination and ankle radiographs according to the Ottawa ankle rules [8–10]. For the purpose of this study, we included only the 170 acute lateral ankle ligament injuries occurred in 148 patients who had been examined within 6 hours of the injury and had no clinical evidence of a syndesmotic injury. All these athletes were managed nonoperatively [11] for the first 48 hours following the injury. This consists of ice application for 15 minutes every hour for the first 6 hours after the examination, and then every 3 hours. The ankle was protected and compressed by the use of elastic bandage, and was kept elevated. We allowed no motion for the first 6 hours, and encouraged isometric exercises of all the periarticular muscles of the ankle thereafter, with active ROM exercises and weight bearing within pain limits.

When reexamined 48 hours after the first assessment, each ankle sprain was classified in the usual fashion, taking into consideration pain, EDE, ability to bear weight, active range of movement, and anterior drawer (AD) and talar tilt (TT) tests. The senior author examined each patient included in the present study. We classified as grade I the patients who had negative clinical tests (AD and TT), as grade II patients with positive AD test, and as grade III those cases with positive AD and TT tests [12].

In addition, on both injured and uninjured side we measured the following:

active ROM by goniometry [13],
ankle EDE with the figure-of-eight method [14,15],
the distance between the posterior articular tip of the tibia to the nearest point of the talus from the AD stress radiographs [16–20].

All patients followed the same rehabilitation protocol, and returned to active sports participation when no symptoms and signs (pain, swelling, tenderness) whatsoever were elicited while training, and the following criteria (compared with the uninjured side) where met:

1. A difference of less than 5° in active ROM
2. A difference of less than 15% in isokinetic strength measured in 60°/s (peroneals, tibialis anterior, gastrocnemius) [21]
3. Negative advanced hop test [22]
4. The latter was the final criterion for return to full athletic activity, and the point of the full rehabilitation time (FRT) we considered for all ankle sprains.

Goniometry

The ankle ROM was measured goniometrically [13]. The goniometer (Lafayette Instrument Company, Lafayette, Indiana) was placed on the lateral maleollus while the patient lay supine. The movable part was parallel to the shaft of the fifth metatarsal, and the unmovable parallel to the fibula (Figs. 1 and 2). The normal ROM is between 20° of dorsiflexion and 50° of plantar flexion [13]. We measured full active ROM bilaterally, calculated the difference, and expressed it as "active ROM deficit."

Edema

The extent of the acute swelling was measured in cm by using the figure-of-eight method (Fig. 3) [14,15]. The measuring tape was applied so that the following landmarks were crossed in a figure-of-eight fashion: (1) navicular tuberosity; (2) the distal tip of the lateral malleolus; (3) the distal tip of the medial malleolus; (4) the base of the fifth metatarsal. The measurement was compared with the uninjured ankle, and expressed it as "EDE difference."

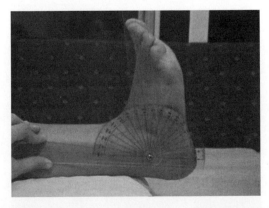

Fig. 1. Goniometric measure of ankle dorsiflexion in an athlete with an acute injury of the lateral ligament complex of the ankle.

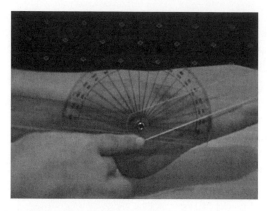

Fig. 2. Goniometric measure of ankle plantar flexion in an athlete with an acute injury of the lateral ligament complex of the ankle.

Stress radiographs

The AD technique was used for the radiographic stress evaluation [16–20] only for grades II and III patients, as in grade I ankle sprains stress radiographs will be nondiagnostic by definition. The heel was supported, while the knee was at 45° of flexion and the foot in neutral to 5° of plantar flexion. A 5-kg sandbag was applied to the anterior aspect of the lower third of tibia (Fig. 4). A lateral radiograph was taken 4 minutes after application of the sandbag, and the same procedure was performed on the uninjured side [18]. We measured the distance between the posterior tip of the articular surface of the tibia and the nearest point of the talus (Fig. 5). A difference greater than 3 mm between uninjured and injured side was considered diagnostic of total ATFL rupture (Figs. 6 and 7) [19,23]. This difference was expressed as "stress radiographs difference."

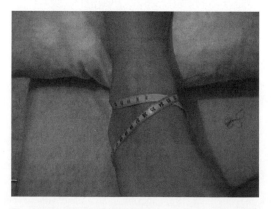

Fig. 3. The figure-of-8 method to measure ankle EDE.

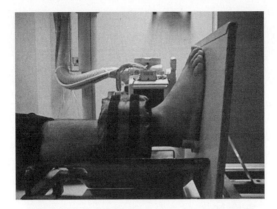

Fig. 4. The apparatus used for AD stress radiographs.

Statistics

Data were entered in a commercially available database, and analyzed using SPSS for Windows, version 8.0 (SPSS, Inc., Chicago, Illinois). Descriptive results are reported as means (SD). MANOVA and Student's t-test were used to compare two groups. Intratester reliability was assessed by intraclass correlation coefficient. Intertester reliability was assessed by the Pearson product moment correlation coefficient. Significance was set at $P \leq 0.05$.

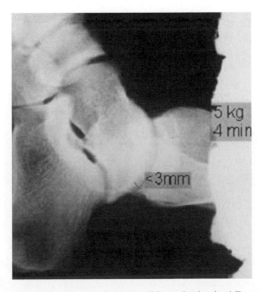

Fig. 5. Measurement of the distance between tibia and talus in AD stress radiographs.

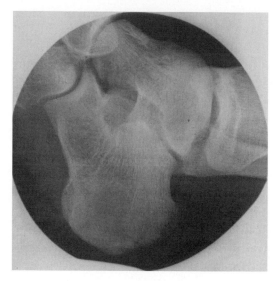

Fig. 6. Normal stress radiographs of uninjured side of a triple jumper with an acute injury of the lateral ligament complex of the ankle.

Results

At the second consultation, 48 hours after the first one, 92 (44.2%) patients were classified as having a grade I sprain, 63 (30.3%) as having a grade II sprain, and 53 (25.5%) as having a grade III sprain (Table 1).

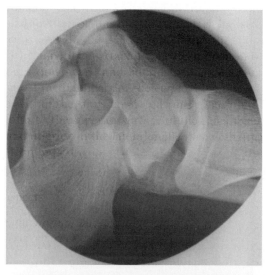

Fig. 7. In the same athlete, stress radiographs revealed a grade IIIB acute injury of the lateral ligament complex of the ankle.

Table 1
Primary classification of ankle injuries in athletes

Grades	No.	%
I	92	44.2
II (anterior drawer test positive)	63	30.3
III (both anterior drawer and talar tilt tests positive)	53	25.5

When we analyzed the stress radiographs results in patients with grade III ankle sprains, 36 patients had a normal AD radiograph test, with a mean difference of 2.19 mm (± 0.75). The remaining 17 patients had a mean difference of 7.41 mm (± 1.54) on the AD radiograph test ($P < 0.01$). Therefore, there are two subgroups in terms of mechanical instability, and this lead us to take a closer look to these subgroups (IIIA and IIIB). The aim was to define their characteristics with the use of objective criteria such as measured active ROM, EDE, and FRT. When full return to sports was considered, we found that all patients with normal AD radiograph test patients (which we called grade IIIA patients) returned to unrestricted athletic activity in a mean time of 30.22 (± 3.3) days. Patients with a side-to-side difference greater than 3 mm on AD radiograph test (which we called grade IIIB patients) returned to unrestricted athletic activity in a mean time of 55.65 (± 4.53) days ($P < 0.01$). There were also significant differences in active ROM between grade IIIA and grade IIIB patients (Table 2).

There were significant differences between the four groups (I, II, IIIA, IIIB) in active ROM, EDE, and FRT, and between patients with grade IIIA and grade IIIB for stress radiographs (Table 3).

Discussion

The value of standard routine radiographs (AP, L, and mortise) in acute ankle sprains is overemphasized. We took AD stress radiographs, as this technique can be performed without the use of complex and expensive devices and is quite painless and precise.

It may be difficult to ascertain the amount of ligamentous damage in patients with acute ankle injuries. The description of the event is generally of no great value: the injury occurs too quickly for patients to accurately recall

Table 2
Results for Grade IIIA and IIIB patients

Grade	IIIA	IIIB	
Active ROM deficit	$14.5 \pm 5.05°$	$21.24 \pm 4.79°$	$P < 0.01$
Edema difference (cm)	2.25 ± 0.37	2.6 ± 0.48	$P < 0.01$
Stress radiograph difference (mm)	2.19 ± 0.75	7.41 ± 1.54	$P < 0.01$
FRT (days)	30.22 ± 3.3	55.65 ± 4.53	$P < 0.01$

Table 3
Results using the revised classification for acute injury of the lateral ligament complex of the ankle

	Clinical tests	Active ROM difference (SD)	Edema difference (SD) (cm)	Stress radiographs (mm)[a] (SD)	FRT (days)[b] (SD)
I		3.96° (2.59)	0.35 (.21)	Not performed	7.24 (1.63)
II	Anterior drawer test positive	8.21° (3.57)	1.58 (.53)	Not performed	14.95 (2.1)
IIIA	Both anterior drawer and talar tilt tests positive	13.92° (4.61)	2.24 (.42)	2.24 (.42)	30.65 (3.07)
IIIB	Both anterior drawer and talar tilt tests positive	20.7° (6.38)	2.57 (.47)	6.81 (1.52)	55.41 (4.92)

[a] $P < 0.01$ between IIIA and IIIB.
[b] $P < 0.01$.

what happened, and the mechanism is frequently similar for all grades of lateral ankle ligament injuries. The site of tear can often be determined by palpating the site of maximal tenderness, and radiographs are necessary to rule out a fracture, as it is difficult to differentiate fracture from severe sprain on clinical grounds. The above variables can make it difficult to classify lateral ankle sprains.

Lateral ankle ligament injuries are graded from I to III [12], based on increasing ligamentous damage and morbidity. In a grade I sprain, the ATFL is stretched with some of the ligament fibers torn, but no frank ligamentous disruption is present. Clinically, the patient presents with mild swelling, little or no hematoma on the lateral aspect ankle, point tenderness on the ATFL, and no or mild restriction of active ROM. Difficulty with full weight bearing is sometimes seen, and there is no laxity on examination. Usually, after appropriate management, the patient suffers no significant functional loss, and returns to sports within 7 to 10 days [12]. A grade II sprain involves a moderate injury to the lateral ligamentous complex, frequently with a complete tear of the ATFL and an additional partial tear of the CFL. Examination shows restricted ROM with localized swelling, echymosis, hemorrhage, and tenderness of the anterolateral aspect ankle. Abnormal laxity may be mild or may not be present. The patient experiences additional functional loss, with inability to toe rise or hop on the injured foot. A Grade II injury may present with swelling and functional loss that makes it indistinguishable from a grade III injury in the acute setting.

A grade III injury implies complete disruption of both the ATFL and CFL, possibly with a capsular tear. An accompanying tear of the posterior talofibular ligament can be present. Examination often reveals diffuse swelling, echymosis on the lateral side of the ankle and heel, and tenderness over the anterolateral capsule, ATFL, and CFL. Moderate to severe laxity to AD or inversion tests is usually present, but may not be elicited, depending on the amount of swelling and muscular spasm during examination.

This anatomic three grade classification is easy to reproduce, but one might need more than 5 days to classify the injury on clinical grounds [24]. ADT and TT tests are subjective and, in early stages, only indicative of the ligamentous integrity [24]. So, although we use them, probably only negative results are reliable, especially in the immediate postinjury period.

High-level athletes demand faster rehabilitation: the typical scenario is of a patient seeking a precise diagnosis and a definite indication of the time needed to return to full sport fitness. MRI scans depict the anatomic integrity of the ligaments, but are expensive, and cannot predict the functional outcome. The method outlined in this study, combined with close follow-up, allows to state with some certainty the length of time that an athlete will require to return to sporting fitness.

In the first instance, we perform a thorough clinical examination of the injured athlete to exclude ankle fractures. The next step is the implementation of PRICE for at least 48 hours, starting just after the injury. When the athlete is examined again 48 hours after the injury, active ROM, EDE, and stress radiographs (if indicated) are assessed. The active ROM, EDE, and stress radiographs protocol can help the examining physician to differentiate acute functional and mechanical instability (grade IIIA and grade IIIB, respectively) and to plan for the management protocol.

The existing classification is not based on clinical and objective measurements. The use of stress radiographs for this purpose is effective, but, to our knowledge, no study was ever performed to correlate it with clinical outcome in terms of returning back to unrestricted sports activities.

The ROM–EDE–stress radiographs (R.E.S) classification that we propose evaluates the severity of lateral ankle injuries, and is an easy and practical method.

We summarize our classification as follows.

In a grade I injury, there are decreased ROM up to 5° compared with the uninjured side, and EDE up to 0.5 cm. In a grade II injury, there are decreased ROM more than 5° and less than 10° degrees, and EDE greater than 0.5 cm and less than 2.0 cm. In a grade IIIA injury, there are decreased ROM greater than 10°, EDE greater than 2.0 cm and normal stress radiographs. Finally, in a grade IIIB injury, there are decreased ROM greater than 10°, EDE greater than 2 cm, and difference in distance between the posterior articular surface of the tibia to the nearest point of talus when comparing uninjured and injured ankles greater than 3 mm (Table 4).

We do not to obtain stress radiographs for grade I and II injuries, making our protocol more practical and cost effective. Also, the use of the AD test is less painful than inversion stressing, and may be repeated without undue pain for the athlete. As the status of the CFL is not outlined by this maneuver, it is important to stress that a complete tear of the ATFL alone is sufficient to fulfil the criteria for subdivision of grade III ankle sprains.

We believe that the initial classification based on clinical criteria, such as clinical tests, pain, and ability to bear weight, is not sufficient for athletes.

Table 4
Revised criteria for the classification of acute injury of the lateral ligament complex of the ankle compared to the uninjured side

Grade	Decreased ROM	Edema	Stress radiographs
I	up to 5°	up to 0.5 cm	Normal
II	5 to 10°	0.5 cm to 2 cm	Normal
IIIA	more than 10°	more than 2 cm	Normal
IIIB	more than 10°	more than 2 cm	Laxity greater than 3 mm

The proposed classification has great value in predicting full return in athletic activities without residual complaints, if the proper rehabilitation program is executed.

References

[1] Brand RL, Collins MF, Templeton T. Surgical repair of ruptured lateral ankle ligaments. Am J Sports Med 1981;9:40–4.
[2] Balduini FC, Vegso JJ, Torg TS, et al. Management and rehabilitation of ligamentous injuries to the ankle. Sports Med 1987;4:364–80.
[3] Botura PM, Bishop JO, Braly G, et al. Acute lateral ankle ligament injuries: a literature review. Foot Ankle 1990;11:107–13.
[4] Bridgman SA, Clement D, Downing A, et al. Population based epidemiology of ankle sprains attending accident and emergency units in the West Midlands of England, and a survey of UK practice for severe ankle sprains. Emerg Med J 2003;20:508–51.
[5] Holmer P, Sondergaard L, Konradsen L, et al. Epidemiology of sprains in the lateral ankle and foot. Foot Ankle Int 1994;15:72–4.
[6] Tropp H, Ascling C, Gillquist J. Prevention of ankle sprains. Am J Sports Med 1985;13(4): 259–62.
[7] Brostrom L. Sprained ankles III. Clinical observations in recent ligament ruptures. Acta Chir Scand 1965;130:560–9.
[8] Stiell IG, Greenberg GH, McKnight RD, et al. Decision rules for the use of radiography in acute ankle injuries: refinement and prospective validation. JAMA 1993;269(9):1127–32.
[9] Papacostas E, Papadopoulos A, Liouliakis C, et al. Validation of Ottawa ankle rules in Greek athletes: a study in the emergency departments of a district general hospital and a sports injuries clinic. Br J Sports Med 2001;35:445–7.
[10] Chande VT. Decision rules for roentgenography of children with acute ankle injuries. Arch Pediatr Adolesc Med 1995;149(3):255–8.
[11] Kannus P, Renstrom P. Treatment for acute tears of the lateral ligaments of the ankle: operation cast or early controlled mobilization. J Bone Joint Surg Am 1991;73:305–12.
[12] Chorley JN, Hergenroeder AC. Management of ankle sprains. Pediatr Ann 1997;26(1): 56–64.
[13] American Academy of Orthopaedic Surgeons. Joint motion. Method of measuring and recording. Chicago: author; 1985.
[14] Diamond JE. Rehabilitation of ankle sprains. Clin Sports Med 1989;8(4):877–89.
[15] Esterson PS. Measurement of ankle joint swelling using a figure of eight. J Orthop Sports Phys Ther 1979;1:51–2.
[16] Grace DL. Lateral ankle ligament injuries. Inversion and anterior stress radiography. Clin Orthop 1984;183:153–9.
[17] Johannsen A. Radiological diagnosis of lateral ligament lesion of the ankle. Acta Ortho Scand 1978;49:295–301.

[18] Lindstrand A, Mortensson W. Anterior Instability in the ankle joint following acute lateral ligamentous sprain. Acta Radiol Diagn (Stockh) 1977;18(5):529–39.

[19] Madner RA. Current methods for the evaluation of ankle ligament injuries. J Bone Joint Surg 1994;76A:1103–11.

[20] Rijke AM. Lateral ankle sprains. Graded stress radiography for accurate diagnosis. Phys Sportsmed 1991;19(2):107–18.

[21] Jacoby S. Isokinetic source book. New York: Biodex Medical Systems; 1997.

[22] Ryan JB. Management of the acute ankle sprain. Clin Sports Med 1989;8(3):477–95.

[23] Renstrom PAFH. Persistently painful sprained ankle. J Am Acad Ortho Surg 1994;2: 270–80.

[24] van Dijk CN, Lim LS, Bossuyt PM, et al. Physical examination is sufficient for the diagnosis of sprained ankles. J Bone Joint Surg 1996;78B:958–62.

ELSEVIER
SAUNDERS

Foot Ankle Clin N Am
11 (2006) 509–519

FOOT AND
ANKLE CLINICS

Scoring Systems for Evaluating Ankle Function

Gideon Mann, MD[a,b,c],*, Meir Nyska, MD[a,b],
Iftach Hetsroni, MD[a,b], Jon Karlsson, MD, PhD[d]

[a]Department of Orthopaedic Surgery, Meir General Hospital, Sapir Medical Center,
59 Tshernichovski St., Kfar-Saba, Israel
[b]Sackler School of Medicine, Tel-Aviv University, P.O. Box 39040,
Ramat Aviv, Tel-Aviv 69978, Israel
[c]The Ribstein Center for Sport Medicine Sciences and Research,
Wingate Institute for Physical Education and Sport, Netanaya 42902, Israel
[d]Department of Orthopaedics, The Sahlgrenska Academy at Göteborg University,
Sahlgrenska University Hospital, SE-416 85 Göteborg, Sweden

In 1975, Good and co-workers [1] published a grading system that was based on four categories (excellent, good, fair, and poor) to evaluate the outcome of ankle injuries. Since then, at least six other scoring scales have been suggested to evaluate the success of conservative management protocols, assess the success of surgical procedures, or evaluate the severity and prognosis of an ankle sprain at the acute stage of injury. The most recent scoring system—probably the only one that was validated fully—was presented by Roos and coworkers [2]. This article discusses various scoring systems that are used to evaluate this pathology.

Function and desirable characteristics

Development of ankle scoring systems is expected as part of the growing accuracy that is required for the evaluation of acute ankle injury management protocols and the various surgical techniques for ankle reconstruction. Realizing their importance in obtaining objective knowledge on the well-being of the previously injured athlete, and in understanding the complexity of success and failure, the authors do not understand why scoring systems had not been developed earlier and why they are used rarely.

---

* Corresponding author. The Regin Medical Center, P.O. Box 3440, Givat Shaul, Jerusalem 91342, Israel.
E-mail address: drmann@regin-med.co.il (G. Mann).

1083-7515/06/$ - see front matter © 2006 Elsevier Inc. All rights reserved.
doi:10.1016/j.fcl.2006.05.001

Scoring systems are devised to combine the various functional, clinical, and objective measurements, and possibly radiographic findings that are used to assess the excellent, good, fair, or poor results of an injury or mode of treatment. A scoring system should include the major findings that determine the result, and only should include sufficient and critical factors to make the scoring system accurate, reliable, and reproducible. Inclusion of too many factors would make the use of the system cumbersome and impractical. The factors that are included should be practical enough to be available for each patient (eg, the system should not include an MRI or a 10-k run), and preferably should be assessed by a health care professional who is not involved in the conservative or surgical management that is being tested. The maximum number of points (10, 20, 50, or 100 points) should be calculated easily and readily.

Scoring systems

Scoring systems for hip [3–6] and knee [6–9] evaluations have been in use for the last 3 decades. An evaluation system for ankle fractures was suggested in the early 1980s [10]. In 1979, Sefton and colleagues [11] used a simple system to evaluate surgically treated unstable ankles based on Good and colleagues [1]. They categorized the results into "excellent," "good," "fair," and "poor" (Table 1).

The first scoring system to evaluate patients whose ankle had undergone surgery following a sprain was devised by St. Pierre and coworkers in 1982 [12], but it failed to gain popularity. St. Pierre and colleagues' system is based on a separate evaluation of activity level, pain, swelling, and functional instability. Each was evaluated as excellent (0), good (1), fair (2), or failure (3) (Table 2).

Scoring system of Karlsson and Peterson, 1991

Karlsson and Peterson [13] published a scoring system in 1991 that was based on eight functional categories: pain, swelling, subjective instability,

Table 1
Sefton scoring scale

Grade 1	Full activity, including strenuous sport
	No pain, swelling or giving way
Grade 2	Occasional aching only after strenuous exercise
	No giving way or feeling of apprehension
Grade 3	No giving way but some remaining apprehension, especially on rough ground
Grade 4	Recurrent instability and giving way in normal activities, with episodes of pain and swelling

From Sefton GK, George J, Filton JM, et al. Reconstruction of the anterior talo-fibular ligament for the treatment of the unstable ankle. J Bone Joint Surg [Br] 1979;61:353; with permission.

Table 2
St Pierre functional scale for evaluation of ankle function after reconstruction

Excellent	Good	Fair	Failure
Level of activity after treatment			
0 - Full return to activity and athletics	1 - Return to full activity with support	2 - Unable to return athletics	3 - Decreased activity
Intensity of pain			
0 - No pain	1 - Mild pain	2 - Moderate pain	3 - Severe pain
Swelling			
0 - No swelling	1 - Swells after exercise	2 - Swells after routine activity	3 - Swells all of the time
Functional instability			
0 - No evidence of instability (no sprains)	1 - Mild instability (1 sprain/y)	2 - Moderate instability (2–3 sprains/y)	3 - Severe instability (greater than 3 sprains/y)

Scale:

Grade of operative repair	*Functional result*
0	excellent
1	good
2–6	fair
>6	failure

From St. Pierre R, Allman F, Bassett III FH, et al. A review of lateral ankle ligamentous reconstructions. Foot ankle 1982;3:114–23; with permission.

stiffness, stair climbing, running, work activities, and use of external support. Each item was allocated a certain number of points, which amounted to a total maximum of 100 points. The scoring scale showed good correlation with a visual analog estimation of ankle function as compiled by the patient, and a good correlation with the functional score of St. Pierre and colleagues, with the talar anterior translation, and with the talar tilt (Table 3).

Scoring system of Mann and coworkers, 1991

In 1991, Mann and coworkers [14–16] developed a scoring system to assess patients who had acute ankle sprains and patients who had undergone surgery for this condition. The system was first used in 1992 in the M.D. thesis of H. Peri [17]. The system emphasizes the functional ability of the athlete while allowing fewer points for purely nonfunctional measurements, such as radiographic findings (tilt and drawer) or range of motion.

The objective measurement portion (36 points) includes the modified Romberg Test, jump from height, figure-eight run, cutting ability, swelling,

Table 3
Karlsson and Peterson scoring system for ankle function

	Degree	Score
Pain	None	20
	During exercise (eg, training)	15
	Walking on uneven surface	10
	Walking on even surface	5
	Constant (severe)	0
Swelling	None	10
	After exercise	5
	Constant	0
Instability (subjective)	None	25
	1–2/y (during exercise)	20
	1–2/mo (during exercise)	15
	Walking on uneven ground	10
	Walking on even ground	5
	Constant (severe) using ankle support	0
Stiffness	None	5
	Moderate (morning, after exercise)	2
	Marked (constant, severe)	0
Stair climbing	No problems	10
	Impaired (instability)	5
	Impossible	0
Running	No problems	10
	Impaired	5
	Impossible	0
Work activities	Same as before injury	15
	Same work, less sports, normal leisure activities	10
	Lighter work, no sports, normal leisure activities	5
	Severely impaired work capacity, decreased leisure activities	0
Support	None	5
	Ankle support during exercise	2
	Ankle support during daily activities	0

Adapted from Karlsson J, Peterson L. Evaluation of ankle joint function: the use of a scoring scale. Foot Ankle Int 1991;1:15–9; with permission.

sensitivity to pressure, drawer test (in millimeters) compared with the other ankle, tilt test (in degrees) compared with the other ankle, dorsiflexion, plantarflexion, varus of heel, and crepitation, for a total of 12 measurements (Table 4a). The functional portion (64 points) includes frequency of recurrent sprain, sports activity, daily activities, walking on a slant, pain, and use of orthopedic supports, with a total of 36 functions (Table 4b). The objective and functional scoring systems have a maximum combined score of 100 points.

The combined scoring system showed a significant correlation with the late occurrence or nonoccurrence of chronic functional instability ($P = .05$). This scoring system is accurate and practical for use in the clinical

Table 4a
Objective scoring system

		Score	1 wk	6 wk	12 wk	6 mo	1 y
Romberg Test modifications (30 s)	No side to side difference (up to 5 s)	9					
	Slight difficulty (5 to 15 s)	4					
	Difficult (over 15 s difference)	0					
Jump 30 cm	Symmetric landing	3					
	Careful at landing	2					
	Lands on one leg	0					
Figure-eight run	Free	3					
	Limited	2					
	Impossible	0					
Cutting	Free	3					
	Limited	2					
	Impossible	0					
Swelling	None	3					
	Mild	2					
	Obvious	0					
Sensitivity	None	3					
	Mild	2					
	Obvious	0					
Drawer	Like other side	2					
	Mild up to 4 mm	1					
	Severe over 4 mm	0					
Tilt	Like other side	2					
	Mild up to 5	1					
	Severe over 5	0					
Dorsiflexion	Like other side	2					
	Loss up to 10	1					
	Loss over 10	0					
Plantarflexion	Like other side	2					
	Loss up to 10	1					
	Loss over 10	0					
Varus of heel	Like other side	2					
	Loss up to 10	1					
	Loss over 10	0					
Crepitation	None	2					
	Mild	1					
	Obvious	0					

The total possible score for the objective scoring system is 36 points.

or research settings for evaluating the outcome of athletes who have been treated conservatively or surgically for ankle sprains.

Scoring system of Kaikkonen and coworkers, 1994

In 1994, Kaikkonen and coworkers [18] published a scoring system that was based on three questions that were chosen after assessment of 11

Table 4b
Functional scoring system

		Score	First visit	6 wk	12 wk	6 mo	1 y
Recurrent sprain	None	28					
	Once in 3 months	20					
	Once in 1 or 2 months	10					
	Once a week/any activity	0					
Sports	Full return as before	10					
	Return at lower level	7					
	Return to noncompetitive sport	4					
	Did not return to sport	0					
Daily activity	Can run on any surface	12					
	Can run only on flat surface	9					
	Can walk but not run on any surface	6					
	Can walk only on flat surface	3					
	Difficulty walking and daily activity	0					
Walking slant 45°	No limitations	5					
	Difficult	3					
	Impossible	0					
Pain	None	5					
	After stressful sports	4					
	After nonstressful sports	3					
	Without physical activity	2					
	Severe and frequent	0					
Orthopedic instrumental use	Not using	4					
	Elastic support only	2					
	Firm (hard) support	0					

The total possible scoring for the functional scoring system is 64 points. The objective and functional scoring systems have a maximum combined score of 100 points.

functional inquiries, two clinical measurements, two strength tests, one functional test, and one balance test. The total number of factors assessed was nine, with a maximum score of 100 points. The researchers found a significant correlation of the system with isokinetic ankle strength, patients' subjective evaluations of their recovery, and patients' subjective functional assessments (Table 5).

Scoring system of de Bie and coworkers, 1997

In 1997, de Bie and coworkers [19] published a scoring system to be used in acute ankle sprains that were not subjected to surgery. The system is based on functional evaluation of pain, stability, weight bearing, swelling,

Table 5
Scoring scale for subjective and functional follow-up evaluation

Questions	Subjective assessment of the injured ankle	
	No symptoms of any kind[a]	15
	Mild symptoms	10
	Moderate symptoms	5
	Severe symptoms	0
	Can you walk normally?	
	Yes	15
	No	0
	Can you run normally?	
	Yes	10
	No	0
Functional test	Climbing down stairs[b]	
	<18 s	10
	18 to 20 s	5
	>20 s	0
Strength tests	Rising on heels with injured leg	
	>40 times	10
	30 to 39 times	5
	<30 times	0
	Rising on toes with injured leg	
	>40 times	10
	30 to 39 times	5
	<30 times	0
Balance test	Single-limb stance with injured leg	
	>55 s	10
	50 to 55 s	5
	<50 s	0
Clinical measurements	Laxity of the ankle joint (ADS)	
	Stable (≤ 5 mm)	10
	Moderate instability (6–10 mm)	5
	Severe instability (>10 mm)	0
	Dorsiflexion range of motion, injured leg	
	>10°	10
	5–9°	5
	<5°	0

Total: excellent = 85–100; good = 70–80; fair = 55–65; poor ≤ 50.

Abbreviation: ADS, anterior drawer sign.

[a] Pain, swelling, stiffness, tenderness, or giving way during activity (mild, only one of these symptoms is present; severe, four or more of these symptoms are present).

[b] Two levels of staircase (length, 12 m) with 44 steps (height, 18 cm; depth, 22 cm).

Adapted from Kaikkonen A, Kannus P, Järvinen M. A performance test protocol and scoring scale for the evaluation of ankle injuries. Am J Sports Med 1994;22:465; with permission.

and the walking pattern, with a maximum obtainable score of 100 points. The system is used to assess the prognosis in acute injuries, and it gave a good correlation with the 4-week outcome in 81% of patients, and with the 2-week outcome in 97% of patients (Table 6).

Table 6
Functional score for assessment of acute lateral ankle sprains (not subjected to surgery) in aim
of anticipating their prognosis

Category	Item	Score
Pain	None	35
	During sports	30
	During running on nonlevel surface	25
	During running on level surface	20
	During walking on nonlevel surface	15
	While carrying load	10
	Constant pain	5
Instability	None	25
	Sometimes during sports (less than once a day)	20
	Frequently during sports (daily)	15
	Sometimes during ADL (less than once a day)	10
	Frequently during ADL (daily)	5
	Every step	0
Weight bearing	Jumping	20
	Standing on toes of injured leg	15
	Standing on injured leg	10
	Standing on two legs	5
	None	0
Swelling	None	10
	Light	6
	Mild	3
	Severe	0
Gait pattern	Running	10
	Normal gait	6
	Mild limp	3
	Severe limp	0

Abbreviation: ADL, activities of daily living.
Adapted from de Bie RA, de Vet HC, van den Wildenberg FA, et al. The prognosis of ankle
sprains. Int J Sports Med 1997;18(4):286; with permission.

Scoring system of Roos and coworkers, 2001

In 2001, Roos and colleagues [2] described the Foot and Ankle Outcome
Score (FAOS). The FAOS is a 42-item questionnaire that assesses patient-
relevant outcomes in five subscales (pain, other symptoms, activities of daily
living, sport and recreation function, and foot and ankle–related quality of
life). This score met all set criteria of validity and reliability, and was judged
to be useful for the evaluation of patient-relevant outcomes related to ankle
ligament injuries (Table 7).

To answer each question, five Likert boxes are used (no, mild, moderate,
severe, extreme). All items are scored from 0 to 4, and each of the five sub-
scale scores is calculated as the sum of the items included. Raw scores are
transformed to a 0 to 100, worst to best, scale. The subscores can be presented graphically as an FAOS profile (Fig. 1) [2].

Table 7
Foot and Ankle Outcome Score

Pain	
P1. How often do you experience foot/ankle pain?	Never, monthly, weekly, daily, always
What amount of pain have you experienced the last week during the following activities?	
P2. Twisting/pivoting on your foot/ankle	None, mild, moderate, severe, extreme
P3. Straightening foot/ankle fully	
P4. Bending foot/ankle fully	
P5. Walking on flat surface	
P6. Going up or down stairs	
P7. At night white in bed	
P8. Sitting or lying	
P9. Standing upright	
Other symptoms	
S1. How severe is your foot/ankle stiffness after first a wakening in the morning?	None, mild, moderate, severe, extreme
S2. How severe is your foot/ankle stiffness after sitting, lying, or resting later in the day?	
Sy1. Do you have swelling in your foot/ankle?	Never, rarely, sometimes, often, always
Sy2. Do you feel grinding, or hear clicking or any other type of noise when your foot/ankle moves?	
Sy3. Does your foot/ankle catch or hang up when moving?	
Sy4. Can you straighten your foot/ankle fully?	Always, often, sometimes, rarely, never
Sy5. Can you bend your foot/ankle fully?	
Activities of daily living	
What difficulty have you experienced in the last week:	
A1. Descending stairs	None, mild, moderate, severe, extreme
A2. Ascending stairs	
A3. Rising from sitting	
A4. Standing	
A5. Bending to floor/pick up an object	
A6. Walking on flat surface	
A7. Getting in/out of car	
A8. Going shopping	
A9. Putting on socks/stockings	
A10. Rising from bed	
A11. Taking off socks/stockings	
A12. Lying in bed (turning over, maintaining foot/ankle position)	
A13. Getting in/out of bath	
A14. Sitting	
A15. Getting on/off toilet	
A16. Heavy domestic duties (eg, moving heavy boxes, scrubbing floors)	
A17. Light domestic duties (eg, cooking, dusting)	

(*continued on next page*)

Table 7 (*continued*)

Sport and recreation function	
What difficulty have you experienced in the last week:	
Sp1. Squatting	None, mild, moderate, severe, extreme
Sp2. Running	
Sp3. Jumping	
Sp4. Turning/twisting on your injured foot/ankle	
Sp5. Kneeling	
Foot and ankle–related quality of life	
Q1. How often are you aware of your foot/ankle problems?	Never, monthly, weekly, daily, always
Q2. Have you modified your life style to avoid potentially damaging activities to your foot/ankle?	Not at all, mildly, moderately, severely, totally
Q3. How much troubled are you with lack of confidence in your foot/ankle?	Not at all, mildly, moderately, severely, extremely
Q4. In general, how much difficulty do you have with your foot/ankle?	None, mild, moderate, severe, extreme

The five answers options are given after each item. If the following items have identical answer options, the answer options are given for the first item only.

The Foot and Ankle Outcome Score (FAOS) and a user's guide can be downloaded at http://www.koos.nu

From Roos EM, Brandsson S, Karlsson J. Validation of the Foot and Ankle Outcome Score for ankle ligament reconstruction. Foot Ankle Int 2001;22(10):790; with permission.

Summary

Each of the seven systems described has advantages and drawbacks that consist of ease or difficulty of application, accuracy, validity, and availability. This article should contribute to make these systems better known and easier to apply, and thus, will encourage their use in clinical practice.

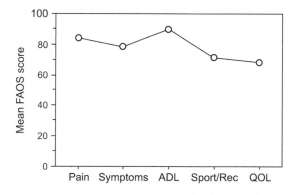

Fig. 1. FAOS profile. Mean score for each of the five FAOS subscales for the study group. ADL, activities of daily living; QOL, foot- and ankle-related quality of life; Sport/Rec, sport and recreation function. (*From* Roos EM, Brandsson S, Karlsson J. Validation of the Foot and Ankle Outcome Score for ankle ligament reconstruction. Foot Ankle Int 2001; 22(10):789; with permission.)

Acknowledgments

The authors would like to express their sincere gratitude to Human Kinetics Publishers, for allowing them to use the material published in the Unstable Ankle: book edited by Nyska & Mann in 2002.

References

[1] Good CJ, Jones MA, Livingstone BN. Reconstruction of the lateral ligament of the ankle. Injury 1975;7:63–5.

[2] Roos EM, Brandsson S, Karlsson J. Validation of the Foot and Ankle Outcome Score for ankle ligament reconstruction. Foot Ankle Int 2001;22(10):788–94.

[3] Anderson G. Hip assessment: a comparison of nine different methods. J Bone Joint Surg Am 1972;54:621–5.

[4] d'Aubigne MD, Postel M. Functional results of hip arthroplasty with acrylic prosthesis. J Bone Joint Surg Am 1954;36:451–75.

[5] Harris WH. Traumatic arthritis of the hip after dislocation and acetabular fractures: treatment by mold arthroplasty. J Bone Joint Surg Am 1969;51:737–54.

[6] Larsson R. Rating sheet for knee function. In: Smillie I, editor. Diseases of the knee joint. Philadelphia: Churchill Livingstone; 1974. p. 29–30.

[7] Lysholm J, Gillqvist J. Evaluation of knee ligament surgery results with special emphasis on use of a scoring scale. Am J Sports Med 1982;10:150–4.

[8] Oretorp N, Gillqvist J, Liljedahl SO. Long-term results of surgery for non-acute anteromedial rotatory instability of the knee. Acta Orthop Scand 1979;50:329–36.

[9] Roos EM, Roos H, Lohmander LS. Knee injury and Osteoarthritis Outcome Score (KOOS). Development of a self-administered outcome measure. J Orthop Sports Phys Ther 1998;78: 88–96.

[10] Olerod C, Molander H. A scoring scale for symptom evaluation after ankle fractures. Arch Orthop Trauma Surg 1984;103:190–4.

[11] Sefton GK, George J, Filton JM, et al. Reconstruction of the anterior talo-fibular ligament for the treatment of the unstable ankle. J Bone Joint Surg [Br] 1979;61:352–4.

[12] St Pierre R, Allman F, Bassett FH III, et al. A review of lateral ankle ligamentous reconstructions. Foot Ankle 1982;3:114–23.

[13] Karlsson J, Peterson L. Evaluation of ankle joint function: the use of a scoring scale. Foot Ankle Int 1991;1:15–9.

[14] Mann G, Elishuv O, Lowe J, et al. Recurrent ankle sprain: literature review. Israel J Sports Med 1994;1:104–8.

[15] Mann G, Elishuv O, Lowe J, et al. Repeated ankle sprain revisited: pathology and pathogenesis. In: Chan KM, Fu F, Maffulli N, et al, editors. Controversies in orthopaedic sports medicine. Baltimore (MD): Williams & Wilkins; 1998. p. 445–9.

[16] Mann G, Nyska M, Matan Y. Scoring systems evaluating ankle function. In: Nyska M, Mann G, editors. The unstable ankle. Champaigne (IL): Human Kinetics; 2002. p. 62–8.

[17] Peri H. Ankle sprain. [MD thesis]. Hadassah-Hebrew University School of Medicine; Jerusalem, Israel: 1992.

[18] Kaikkonen A, Kannus P, Järvinen M. A performance test protocol and scoring scale for the evaluation of ankle injuries. Am J Sports Med 1994;22:462–9.

[19] de Bie RA, de Vet HC, van den Wildenberg FA, et al. The prognosis of ankle sprains. Int J Sports Med 1997;18(4):285–9.

ELSEVIER
SAUNDERS

Foot Ankle Clin N Am
11 (2006) 521–530

FOOT AND
ANKLE CLINICS

Management of Acute Ligament Injuries of the Ankle

Jon Karlsson, MD, PhD*, Michael Sancone, MD

*Department of Orthopaedics, Sahlgrenska University Hospital, Göteborg University,
SE-416 85 Göteborg, Sweden*

Ligament injuries to the lateral ankle ligaments have in several studies been shown to be the most common sports-related injuries [1–3], accounting for approximately 25% of all sports-related injuries. Their incidence is approximately 5000 injuries per day in the United Kingdom, and 23,000 in the United States [2,4,5]. Patients with ankle sprain constitute 7% to 10% of all those examined in emergency departments in Scandinavia [2]. These studies are, however, more than 10 years old, and more recent information has implied that the risk of ankle ligament injuries is lower than previously anticipated. In a recent study, Bridgman and colleagues [6] found that the incidence rates for ankle sprain cases attending accident and emergency departments were somewhat lower than previously reported. The incidence rate was 60.9 per 10 000, with remarkable age and sex differences. Of all injuries, 14% were classified as severe. An elasticated preshaped compression stocking was used routinely as treatment in 55% of the patients, while immobilization using cast or brace was used in only 5%. These authors concluded that there was a wide variation in the management of severe ankle sprains, and, in fact, most patients were managed with minimal mechanical support.

Beynnon and colleagues [7] found that the incidence rate of first-time inversion ankle ligament trauma was less than 1 per 1000 days of exposure to sport, again a value lower than what was previously reported. These researchers found that ankle injuries were associated with the type of sport among females, with the risk highest in female basketball. The relative risk was slightly higher for women than men [7].

Despite the high number of injuries, management remains controversial. Traditionally, acute ankle ligament injuries have been divided into Grade I, II, and III, depending on the amount of soft-tissue injury, bleeding, and

---

* Corresponding author.
E-mail address: jon.karlsson@vgregion.se (J. Karlsson).

1083-7515/06/$ - see front matter © 2006 Elsevier Inc. All rights reserved.
doi:10.1016/j.fcl.2006.07.008

functional impairment [2,4,5]. This distinction is, however, arbitrary, and very seldom used in clinical practice. Some researches advocate early mobilization for all types of injuries, while others manage Grade III ligament injuries with cast immobilization or even surgical repair [8]. Most scientific evidence favors functional management. Despite the extremely high number of injuries, there are surprisingly few well conducted (level I) studies. After reviewing 12 prospective studies where functional management was compared with cast immobilization and surgical repair, Kannus and Renström showed that functional management produced equal results or better compared with the other two management methods, without the increased risk of complications [2].

Although many authors advocate early mobilization, the scientific evidence is somewhat scanty. The best studies on acute injuries are summarized in three Cochrane reviews: more high-quality studies are needed, and none of the reviews is really conclusive [9–11].

Acute ligament injuries

Early diagnosis, functional management, and rehabilitation are the keys to prevention of chronic ligament instability of the ankle. Verhagen and colleagues [12] reviewed current data concerning the efficacy of preventive measures on the incidence of ankle ligament injuries. The use of either tape or brace reduced the incidence of ankle sprains. Moreover, the use of tape or brace resulted in less severe ankle sprain. Also, braces were more effective than tape in preventing ankle sprains. The effect of shoes was controversial. Contrary to what is believed by most researchers, it was not clear which athletes benefited most from the use of preventive measures: those with previous injury, or those without. Braces appeared to be more effective only in athletes with previous ankle sprains. Also, proprioceptive training reduces the incidence of ankle sprains both in athletes with recurrent ankle sprains equally and in those without any history of ankle sprain. Without doubt, prevention should be highlighted and studied on a larger scale, using randomized study design.

The on-field management of fresh injuries relies on the RICE principle [2]. The most vulnerable of the lateral ligaments is the anterior talofibular ligament, followed by a combined rupture of this ligament and the calcaneofibular ligament [1,3]. Other injuries, such as injuries to the deltoid ligament, are much less frequent, and occur with a frequency of less than 10% of all injuries. Prevention of ligament injuries has gained much attention recently: approximately 75% of all injuries are recurrences, and may thus potentially be prevented, provided that a sound protocol being used [13–15]. Prevention by either coordination training using balance boards or by external support can significantly reduce the number of ligament injuries. Ankle tape or functional splinting, proficiently completed by the use of an Air-Stirrup pneumatic splint, are preferred by many athletes. Boyce and colleagues

[16] compared the elastic support bandage and Air-Cast ankle brace in a randomized controlled trial. Of the 50 patients enrolled into the study; 35 completed the trial. The Air-Cast ankle brace (Fig. 1) for lateral ankle ligament sprains produced a significant improvement in ankle joint function (assessment by the modified Karlsson scoring scale), at both 10 days and 1 month, compared with an elastic support bandage.

A few studies have compared early mobilization with cast immobilization. Prins [17] compared early mobilization to 3-week immobilization, and found that there were no significant differences in any outcome variable. Brakenbury and Kotowski [18] compared early mobilization and 1-week immobilization. These researchers found that early mobilization was superior in terms of functional outcome. However, they included only minor injuries, and the follow-up was far from complete. Brooks and colleagues [19] showed that early mobilization including physiotherapy was superior to no management, soft-bandage external support, and immobilization (treatment time varied). Eiff and colleagues [20] compared early mobilization with 10-day immobilization, and found that early mobilization produced better short-term results, but no difference in the long term. In the study by Zwipp and colleagues [21], 189 patients were randomly allocated to cast immobilization for 5 weeks, functional brace for 5 weeks, or primary surgical repair followed by cast immobilization for 5 weeks. Identical rehabilitation protocol was used after the first 5 weeks. Patients undergoing functional bracing had better outcome than those immobilized in a cast. There were no differences in terms of laxity measurements between any of the groups. The surgically managed patients did equally well as the two other groups,

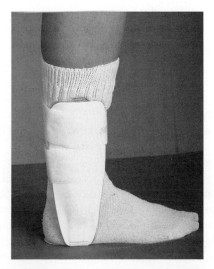

Fig. 1. The Aircast Air-Stirrup(r) ankle brace (viewed from the side) is often used with success in the acute phase treatment.

but were not superior in any functional outcome measure. At 24 months, there were no differences between any of the groups in terms of radiographic measurement of laxity, range of motion, and patient satisfaction.

A classical study on surgical management was conducted by Broström [3], who showed superior results in patients undergoing surgery. However, he also showed satisfactory results in patients managed with early mobilization. His conclusion was that functional management should therefore be preferred, as surgery would lead to many patients undergoing an operation without needing it, with increased risk of complications. Korkala and colleagues [22] compared acute surgical management with early mobilization (elastic bandage) and cast immobilization. In that study, 150 patients were randomly allocated to three groups, but less than 100 were followed for 2 years or more. Recurrent sprains occurred in approximately 20% of the patients in all groups, and there were no differences in terms of functional outcome, as well as radiographic laxity measurements, such as talar tilt (TT) and anterior talar translation (ATT). Kaikkonen and colleaguse [23] compared primary surgical repair combined with early mobilization to early controlled mobilization alone in a prospective study. The follow-up was only 9 months. Excellent/good results were achieved in 87% of patients undergoing functional management, and in 60% of the patients undergoing surgery, respectively. Early mobilization produced better results than surgery combined with mobilization. None of the above-mentioned studies strongly favors early surgery. On the contrary, early functional management, especially mobilization, seems to be the most favorable management.

Stress radiographs

One important question arises concerning the use stress radiography in the diagnosis of acute ankle ligament injuries. The methods most employed are measurements of TT and ATT. Clinicians have often relied on the TT and ATT values to diagnose both acute and chronic ligament insufficiency. Either manual techniques or mechanical devices are used. One major problem is the fact that there is a significant variability in the values defined as normal for both TT and ATT. Values have varied between 4 and 10 mm of ATT, or >1 to 3 mm compared with the contralateral (healthy) side, and 7° to 11°. The conclusion drawn from existing studies is that stress radiographs are not useful, at least in the diagnostic evaluation of acute injuries. One major reason for this is many studies suggest that ligament laxity after acute rupture is not strongly correlated to the development of late symptoms [2,24]. There might be a place for stress radiographs in terms of chronic ligament insufficiency, but their role is still much debated (see other articles in the present issue).

Surgical repair

There is no major place for surgical repair after acute ligament ruptures [25–27]. After a rehabilitation program consisting of functional management, active range-of-motion exercises, coordination training, peroneal strengthening, and early weight bearing, the functional results are excellent or good in 70% to 90% of patients, while 10% to 30% of patients develop secondary symptoms of chronic instability or pain [24,25,27]. Probably, early weight bearing is the cornerstone of early functional management. However, even though there is substantial evidence to suggest that early mobilization with active rehabilitation is probably the management of choice, there are only a few randomized, controlled studies comparing different management modalities [27,28]. In a recent meta-analysis, no management of lateral ankle ligament ruptures led to an increased number of residual symptoms [29]. Surgical management produced better outcome than functional management. On the other hand, functional management was superior to cast immobilization for 6 weeks. Surgery was associated with higher costs, as well as increased risk of complications, such as wound-healing problems, nerve damage, and possibly infections. A recent Cochrane review showed that functional management is the most favorable strategy for acute ankle ligament injuries, at least when compared with immobilization [11]. Concerning surgical versus nonsurgical management for acute injuries of the lateral ligament complex, there is insufficient scientific evidence from randomized, controlled studies to determine the relative effectiveness of surgical and conservative management of these injuries, according to a second Cochrane review [8]. This might imply that surgical management is not superior to any other management. It is also obvious that, following failed conservative management, late reconstructive procedures can be performed with satisfactory results, even several years after the initial injury [11]. Here, procedures, such as anatomic reconstructions come into play, and several studies have shown excellent or good results in the majority of patients (approximately 90%), with low risk of complications.

Functional management

The extent of injury, that is, being Grade I, II, or III, might play an important role. Two prospective randomized studies have evaluated the effect of early range-of-motion training, full early weight bearing, combined with either Air-Cast stirrup or specially designed compression pads [27]. Both studies showed that early functional management resulted in significantly shorter sick leave, and facilitated earlier return to sports, without the risk of inferior functional results in the long run. One of theses studies showed that the mean sick leave was shortened from 10.2 days to 5.6 days, and the return to sports from 19 to 9 days with functional management using specially designed compression pads for the first 24 hours, elevation of the injured foot (24 hours), repeated elastic wrapping, that is, compression bandage, followed by ankle tape, early full weight bearing (no crutches), and proprioceptive range-of-motion training. There were no complications, and the risk of residual instability was not increased. One Cochrane review compared different functional management strategies for the management of acute ankle ligament injuries. This study showed that the use of elastic bandage was correlated to fewer complications than tape, but, on the other hand, was associated with slower return to work and sport. Semirigid ankle braces produced less ankle laxity than elastic bandages. Lace-up ankle support was found to be more effective, especially in reducing swelling in the short term compared with semirigid braces, elastic bandage, and tape. Thus, either semirigid brace or lace-up support should probably be preferred, even though the total evidence is not strong [11]. Moreover, early weight training, combined with range-of-motion training, is beneficial. The general principle is that the early rehabilitation is the mainstay of management. Immobilization should probably never be used, not even in case of Grade III injury, even though the literature is somewhat controversial on this issue [28,29]. Several studies compare immobilization and early mobilization, and none favor immobilization in terms of better outcome [30]. Moreover, immobilization may result in joint stiffness, muscle atrophy, and loss of proprioception.

The long-term prognosis is most probably not altered by early functional training [7]. Studies have shown that the best external support is strong evertor muscles. Therefore, a combination of isokinetic strength training with proprioception training will shorten rehabilitation, and serve as secondary prophylaxis [31,32]. However, functional instability is a complex syndrome, and there are several factors at play, such as increased laxity, proprioceptive deficit, and peroneal muscle weakness, either alone or most often in combination.

Rehabilitation

In the acute phase, the main objective is pain relief, but, as soon as possible after the injury, management is aimed at restoring range of motion, without loss of proprioception [33,34]. Rehabilitation can be divided into four phases, namely initial, early rehabilitation, late rehabilitation, and functional phases. The length of each phase depends on each individual's healing capabilities. The initial phase is directed at reduction of swelling, often using compression bandage, but also sometimes using anti-inflammatory medication, 1 or 2 days of rest, ice, and elevation, that is, the general RICE principle. Sometimes, ultrasound and electrotherapy are added, but their beneficial effect has not been confirmed in any controlled study [35]. Not to lose neuromuscular coordination, gait training, including early weight bearing and balance-board training, is started as early as possible. Full weight bearing is probably one of the most important aspects of early rehabilitation. This initial phase lasts in most instances approximately 1 week after the injury. In weeks 2 to 4, rehabilitation is aimed at restoring normal range of motion of the ankle, with active exercises. Sometimes, manual therapy and kinetotherapy are added, but again, there is no convincing evidence [36]. Passive movement of the ankle joint can be used to increase the range of motion in the sagittal plane. Stretching of the calf muscles is important to increase dorsiflexion. Tilt or balance-board exercises are increased, both in terms of time and intensity. Training is first aimed at balance on both legs, and thereafter on one (the injured one) leg. Cryotherapy is often continued during this phase. Anti-inflammatory medication may be used, as inflammation is often persisting. The athlete is allowed to return to sports activities, provided an external support is continuously used, such as an ankle tape or brace [37–40].

The late rehabilitation phase is usually reached approximately around week 5, and the weight-bearing exercises should be increased [41]. The main goal of this phase is training of muscular strength, endurance, and neuromuscular function. The final functional phase starts around week 9. Return to full sports activity, including jumping, turning, and twisting, should be completed. External support should always be used during the entire functional phase, to reduce the risk of recurrence of the ankle sprain. Supervised protocols can be used both after acute first-time injury and in chronic or recurrent ankle insufficiency. Foot orthoses are often used, although the scientific evidence is limited [42–45].

Before deciding on surgical management in chronically unstable ankles, a well-planned rehabilitation protocol should be completed. This protocol is based on isokinetic strength training of the peroneal muscles, and proprioceptive training. The goal of the protocol is to decrease weakness of the peroneal muscles, and to regain normal proprioceptive function and protective reflexes. The last few weeks of the rehabilitation program should always concentrate on sports activity.

Prevention

The best way to manage ligament injuries is to prevent them. Although this is practically impossible, it is probable that many such injuries might, in fact, be prevented. There are two main methods, both of which have been proven successful in clinical practice, and there is some evidence to support both methods, namely proprioceptive training and external ankle support [40,46]. There is, however, little scientific evidence, to support the preventive effect, especially in terms of ankle taping. Some studies have shown that balance-board training will reduce the risk of ankle ligament injuries, especially in those with previous injuries. The effect, however, is either less pronounced or unknown in athletes with previously uninjured ligaments. In other words, the important question whether the first-time ligament injury can be prevented using proprioceptive training has yet to be answered [37,40]. The second method is the use of external ankle support, either ankle tape or brace. There is very little evidence for the use of ankle tape, and the mechanism behind the function of ankle tape is not well understood [37]. Several studies suggested that tape may reduce ankle laxity, limit the extremes of ankle motion, or shorten the reaction time of the peroneal muscles, thereby affecting the proprioceptive function of the ligaments and the joint capsule. But, as the tape becomes loose after 15 to 30 minutes of use, it has never been proven how it really works. Despite this, ankle tape is commonly used in clinical practice and is preferred by many athletes and athletic trainers. There is more evidence for the use of ankle braces, especially the semirigid Air-stirrup brace [40]. A combination of different exercises and modalities should probably be used. Ankle disk training or semirigid ankle brace appear to the most effective methods for this purpose.

Summary

Ligament injuries of the ankle are common and troublesome. Management may seem easy, but residual symptoms are common. Grade III injuries still generate controversy in terms of the best management available, and more studies are needed when it comes to early mobilization, cast immobilization, or surgery. Even the three Cohrane reviews published to date are not conclusive.

References

[1] Balduini FC, Vegso JJ, Torg JS, et al. Management and rehabilitation of ligamentous injuries of the ankle. Sports Med 1987;4:364–80.
[2] Kannus P, Renström P. Treatment for acute tears of the lateral ligaments of the ankle. Current concepts review. J Bone Joint Surg 1991;73-A:305–12.
[3] Broström L. Sprained ankles. A pathologic, arthrographic, and clinical study. Dissertation, Karolinska Institute, Stockholm; 1966.
[4] Karlsson J. Chronic lateral instability of the ankle joint. A clinical, radiological and experimental study. Dissertation, Göteborg University, Sweden; 1989.
[5] Lynch SA, Renström PAFH. Treatment of acute lateral ankle ligament rupture in the athlete: conservative versus surgical treatment. Sports Med 1999;9:61–71.
[6] Bridgman SA, Clement D, Downing A, et al. Population based epidemiology of ankle sprains attending accident and emergency units in the West Midlands of England, and a survey of UK practice for severe ankle sprains. Emerg Med J 2003;20:508–10.
[7] Beynnon BD, Vacek PM, Murphy D, et al. First-time inversion ankle ligament trauma. The effect of sex, level of competition, and sport on the incidence of injury. Am J Sports Med 2005;33:1485–91.
[8] Kaikkonen A, Hyppänen E, Kannus P, et al. Long-term functional outcome after primary repair of the lateral ligaments of the ankle. Am J Sports Med 1997;25:150–5.
[9] Kerkoffs GMMJ, Struijs PAA, Marti RK, et al. Different functional treatment strategies for acute lateral ankle ligament injuries in adults. Cochrane Database Syst Rev 2002;3: CD002938.
[10] Kerkoffs GMMJ, Handoll HHG, de Bie R, et al. Surgical versus conservative treatment for acute injuries of the lateral ligament complex of the ankle in adults. Cochrane Database Syst Rev 2002;3:CD000380.

[11] Kerkoffs GMMJ, Rowe BH, Assendelft WJJ, et al. Immobilisation and functional treatment for acute lateral ankle ligament injuries in adults. Cochrane Database Syst Rev 2002;3: CD003762.

[12] Verhagen EALM, van Mechelen W, de Vente W. The effect of preventive measures on the incidence of ankle sprains. Critical review. Clin J Sports Medicine 2000;10:291–6.

[13] Asthon-Miller JA, Ottaviani RA, Hutchinson C. What best protects the inverted weight-bearing ankle against further inversion. Am J Sports Med 1996;24:800–9.

[14] Eils E, Rosenbaum D. A multi-station proprioceptive exercise program in patients with ankle instability. Med Sci Sports Exerc 2001;33:1991–8.

[15] Glick JM, Gordon RB, Nishimoto D. The prevention and treatment of ankle injuries. Am J Sports Med 1976;4:136–41.

[16] Boyce SH, Quigley MA, Campbell S. Management of ankle sprains: a randomised controlled trial of the treatment of inversion injuries using an elastic support bandage or an Aircast ankle brace. Br J Sports Med 2005;39:91–6.

[17] Prins JG. Diagnosis and treatment of injury to the lateral ligament of the ankle. Acta Chir Scand 1978;486:3–149.

[18] Brakenbury PH, Kotowski J. A comparative study of the management of ankle sprains. Br J Clin Pract 1983;37:181–5.

[19] Brooks SC, Potter BT, Rainey JB. Treatment for partial tears of the lateral ligament of the ankle: a prospective trial. BMJ 1981;282:606–7.

[20] Eiff MP, Smith AT, Smith GE. Early mobilization versus immobilization in the treatment of lateral ankle sprains. Am J Sports Med 1994;22:83–8.

[21] Zwipp H, Hoffman R, Thermann H, et al. Rupture of the ankle ligaments. Int Orthop 1991; 15:245–9.

[22] Korkala O, Rusanen M, Jokipii P, et al. A prospective study of the treatment of severe tears of the lateral ligament s of the ankle. Int Orthop 1987;11:13–7.

[23] Kaikkonen A, Kannus P, Järvinen M. Surgery versus funtional treatment in ankle ligament tears. Clin Orthop Relat Res 1996;326:19–22.

[24] Freeman MAR, Dean MRE, Hanham IWF. The etiology and prevention of functional instability of the foot. J Bone Joint Surg 1965;47-B:678–85.

[25] Karlsson J, Lansinger O. Lateral instability of the ankle joint. Clin Orthop Relat Res 1992; 276:253–61.

[26] Karlsson J, Lansinger O, Faxén E. Conservative treatment of chronic lateral instability of the ankle. Swedish Med J 1991;88:1404–6.

[27] Karlsson J, Eriksson BI, Swärd L. Early functional treatment for acute ligament injuries of the ankle joint. Scand J Med Sci Sports 1996;6:341–5.

[28] Karlsson J, Faxén E, Eriksson BI. Ankle joint ligament injuries: prevention, evaluation and treatment. Crit Rev Phys Rehabil Med 1996;8:183–200.

[29] Pijenburg ACM, van Dijk CN, Bossuyt PMM, et al. Treatment of ruptures of the lateral ankle ligaments: a meta-analysis. J Bone Joint Surg 2000;82-A:761–73.

[30] Vaes PH, Duquet W, Castelyn PP. Static and dynamic roentgenographic analysis of ankle stability in braced and non-braced stable and functionally unstable ankles. Am J Sports Med 1998;26:692–702.

[31] Konradsen L, Ravn JB. Ankle instability caused by prolonged reaction time. Acta Orthop Scand 1990;61:388–90.

[32] Mascaro TB, Swanson LE. Rehabilitation of the foot and ankle. Orthop Clin North Am 1994;25:147–60.

[33] Lephart SM, Pincivero DM, Giraldo JL. The role of proprioception in the management and rehabilitation of athletic injuries. Am J Sports Med 1997;25:130–7.

[34] Matsuaka N, Yokoyama S, Tsurusaki T. Effect of ankle disk training combined with tactile stimulation to the leg and foot on functional instability of the ankle. Am J Sports Med 2001; 29:25–30.

[35] Makuloluwe RTB, Mouxas GL. Ultrasound in the treatment of sprained ankles. Practioner 1977;218:586–8.

[36] Karlsson J, Andréasson GO. The effect of external ankle support in chronic lateral ankle joint instability. An electromyographic study. Am J Sports Med 1992;20:257–61.

[37] Raikin SM, Parks BG, Noll KH. Biomechanical evaluation of the ability of casts and brace to immobilize the ankle and hindfoot. Foot Ankle Int 2001;22:214–9.

[38] Stover CN. Air-Stirrup management of ankle injuries in the athlete. Am J Sports Med 1980; 8:360–5.

[39] Simpson KJ, Cravens S, Higbie E. A comparison of the Sport Stirrup, Malleoloc, and Swede-O ankle orthoses for the foot ankle kinematics of a rapid lateral movement. Int J Sports Med 1999;20:396–402.

[40] Zöch C, Fialka-Moser V, Quitton M. Rehabilitation of ligamentous ankle injuries: a review of recent studies. Br J Sports Med 2003;37:291–5.

[41] Uh BS, Beynnon BD, Helie BV. The benefit of a single-leg strength training program for the muscles around the untrained ankle. Am J Sports Med 2000;28:568–73.

[42] Hertel J, Denegar CR, Buckely WE. Effect of rear foot orthototics on postural sway after lateral ankle sprain. Arch Phys Med Rehabil 2001;82:1000–3.

[43] Löfvenberg R, Kärrholm J. The influence of an ankle orthosis on the talar and calcaneal motions in chronic lateral instability of the ankle. Am J Sports Med 1993;21:224–30.

[44] Nester CJ, Hutchins S, Bowker P. Effect of foot orthoses on rear foot complex cinematics during walking gait. Foot Ankle Int 2001;22:133–9.

[45] Stacoff A, Reinschmidt C, Nigg BM. Effects of foot orthoses on skeletal motion during running. Clin Biomech (Bristol, Avon) 2000;15:54–64.

[46] Sheth P, Yu B, Laskowski ER. Ankle disk training influences reaction time of selected muscles in a simulated ankle sprain. Am J Sports Med 1997;25:538–43.

ELSEVIER
SAUNDERS

Foot Ankle Clin N Am
11 (2006) 531–537

FOOT AND
ANKLE CLINICS

Conservative Management of Chronic Ankle Instability

Adam Ajis, MBBS, MRCSEd,
Nicola Maffulli, MD, MS, PhD, FRCS (Orth)*

*Department of Trauma and Orthopaedic Surgery, Keele University School of Medicine,
Thornburrow Drive, Hartshill, Stoke on Trent ST4 7QB Staffs, United Kingdom*

The mechanism of injury of lateral ankle sprains is usually a forced inversion injury with the tibiotalar joint in plantar flexion. Up to 20% of lateral ankle sprains progress to functional instability [1].

Inversion injuries of the ankle account for up to 25% of all musculoskeletal injuries [2]. Despite the high incidence, there is still some contention about the optimal method of management. Proposed management modalities include surgical repair/reconstruction, rigid/semirigid casting, bracing, elastic bandaging, strapping, ultrasound, temperature contrast baths, electric current therapy, hyperbaric oxygen, oral anti-inflammatories, oral proteolytic enzymes, and injectable steroids [3]. These options are usually combined with rest, compression, ice, and elevation. Conservative management involves one or more of the above modalities within a program of either strict immobilization or early controlled movement and rehabilitation [3]. This article discusses some of the conservative management modalities described in the literature.

Types of instability

Two types of ankle instability are described, namely functional and mechanical. Mechanical instability is abnormal laxity of the ligamentous restraints, and is a sign. Functional instability refers to abnormal function, with recurrent episodes of the ankle giving way, and is a symptom. The two types of instability can exist independently of one another, but often occur together. Indeed, a patient can have minimal mechanical instability

---

* Corresponding author.
E-mail address: n.maffulli@keele.ac.uk (N. Maffulli).

1083-7515/06/$ - see front matter © 2006 Elsevier Inc. All rights reserved.
doi:10.1016/j.fcl.2006.07.004　　　　　　　　　　　　　*foot.theclinics.com*

(ie, minimal laxity) and report giving way, that is, functional instability. Therefore, the terms "laxity" and "instability" should not be used synonymously.

Clinical features

Anatomy

In neutral position, the tight fit of the talus between the tibia and fibula stabilize the ankle joint [4]. The compressive loads imposed under weight bearing enhance osseous stability [4]. With increasing plantar flexion, the osseous constraints are lessened, and the soft tissues are more susceptible to strain and injury [4].

The lateral ankle joint ligamentous complex consists primarily of three structures: the anterior talofibular ligament (ATFL), the calcaneofibular ligament (CFL), and the posterior talofibular ligament (PTFL) (Fig. 1).

The ATFL is the most anterior structure, and is the weakest and most easily injured of these ligaments [5]. The ATFL is often described as a thickening of the lateral joint capsule [6]. When the foot is plantar flexed, the ATFL is vertical, and is the primary stabilizing structure of the ankle during an inversion stress.

The CFL is a round, cord-like extracapsular structure that originates from the inferior distal surface of the fibula, extends posteroinferiorly, deep to the peroneal tendons, and attaches on a small tubercle on the posterior aspect of the lateral calcaneal surface. The CFL is vertical when the

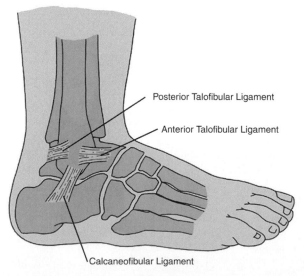

Fig. 1. The ligamentous complex of the lateral aspect of the ankle.

foot is dorsiflexed, when it becomes the primary ankle stabilizer and secondary subtalar joint stabilizer. Isolated injuries of the CFL are rare.

The PTFL is the strongest and least vulnerable of the three ligaments; isolated ruptures are extremely rare. It is most commonly injured in severe ankle sprains after the ATFL and CFL have been disrupted. It is a trapezoid-shaped structure, which originates from the distal portion of the digital fossa of the fibula and inserts on the posterolateral tubercle of the talus, and on the os trigonum when present.

History

Most patients give a clear history of one or more ankle injuries. However, some patients, especially those with varus or cavovarus foot, may develop symptoms of ankle instability without injury [3]. Typically, patients complain of repeated giving way of the ankle. Swelling and pain may accompany giving way, which is often commoner on slopes or uneven ground.

Examination

It is important to identify the underlying causes of instability. In particular, the overall foot shape should be evaluated, looking particularly for hindfoot varus, and adequate neurologic examination should be performed. The shoes will give information on heel contact. Generalized joint laxity should be sought.

Tenderness is usually maximal over the lateral ligament, often over the ATFL only. A few patients, normally those with more complex injuries, also have localized tenderness over the deltoid ligament. Some patients have rather generalized joint line tenderness, palpable synovitis, or an effusion. Tenderness or swelling over the Achilles, peroneal, or tibialis posterior tendons should be identified. There is an association between ankle instability and peroneal tendon instability: patients will usually complain of snapping or giving way over the peroneal tendons, and instability is maximal on plantar flexion and eversion.

Laxity is demonstrated with the anterior draw and tilt tests. The anterior draw test should be performed with the ankle in 20° of plantar flexion [7]. The tibia may be pushed posteriorly against the fixed foot, or the foot can be drawn forward. The characteristic positive sign is a "suction sign," as the synovium is sucked into the joint, drawing the skin inward in the lateral gutter. However, in many patients there is no suction sign, but the talus can obviously be drawn anteriorly more than on the contralateral side. Tohyama and colleagues [8] showed in cadavers that 30 N force produced more difference in displacement between injured and normal sides than 60 N.

The talar tilt test is conventionally performed by tilting the hindfoot and looking for a suction sign or asymmetric movement. The ankle should be in physiologic plantar flexion [7]. Palpation of the talar neck will assist in differentiating between movement in the ankle and the subtalar joint.

There may well be no great correlation between mechanical stability (ie, laxity) and functional stability. Therefore, a patient may present with great laxity, and report no or very little instability. In these patients, the role of surgery is dubious, and conservative management is probably a safe option.

Imaging

Plain anteroposterior and lateral radiographs of the ankle are generally obtained to evaluate the joint and ascertain the presence of associated injuries. Obtaining these films with the patient standing allows accurate assessment of joint space and alignment. In patients with cavus or cavovarus feet, a standing hindfoot alignment view can be done, which differentiates between malalignment within and below the ankle [9]. Standing lateral and dorsoplantar views of the foot allow further evaluation of possible associated deformity.

Stress radiography is the "gold standard" for detecting mechanical ankle instability. However, there has been wide variation in the criteria for diagnosing instability. Karlsson and colleagues [10] performed a most comprehensive study, establishing criteria for radiographic instability of an anterior draw of 10 mm or more, or a talar tilt of 9° or more. If an opposite stable ankle was available for comparison, an anterior draw of 3 mm or a talar tilt of 3° more than the other side would be significant. However, as the management of acute ankle sprains is based on functional nonoperative modalities, and does not depend on the degree of ankle instability on stress views, stress radiographs have no clinical relevance in the acute situation. In cases of functional instability, the large variability in both injured and noninjured ankles precludes their routine use [11].

Magnetic resonance imaging may be used in preoperative planning if doubts still persist.

Conservative management

Most studies on surgery for chronic ankle instability comment that "the patients had full nonsurgical management before being considered for surgery": this is considered good practice [12,13].

However, only one published series examined the effect of functional rehabilitation on chronic instability. Karlsson [14] found that 50% of patients with chronic instability benefited from a structured rehabilitation program. Patients with mechanical instability were less likely to benefit than those with purely functional instability.

Modalities

Conservative management of patients with functional ankle instability follows the paradigm typical of acute management of soft tissue injuries, using the RICE principles. Peroneal strengthening, proprioceptive training, lateral heel wedges, bracing and strapping are the main modalities of ankle rehabilitation [15–17]. Lateral heel wedges and Achilles tendon stretching are helpful in preventing hindfoot malpositioning that leaves lateral ligaments prone to injury [18]. Proprioceptive training and peroneal strengthening work by stabilizing the ankle and hindfoot through improvement in maintaining ankle position when external forces are applied to it. After proprioceptive training, patients are less likely to allow the ankle to adopt a position that makes it more vulnerable to injury [17–19]. Proprioception training can be performed using an ankle tilt board [20]. Improved ankle proprioception leads to better dynamic ankle joint stability, and has a protective role against future sprains [21].

Peroneal muscle reaction times were significantly longer in patients with ankle instability [19]. Patients probably recruit their peroneal musculature slightly later, and cannot protect themselves from further inversion and injury. The same study found that training, taping, and external immobilization work to restrict the extremes of motion and shorten peroneal muscle reaction time. This was not statistically significant [19].

Ankle braces have been widely used to compensate for instability. Those braces that provide adequate support clinically tend to be too bulky, and are thus unpopular with athletes [22]. Aircast (UCBL, Summit, New Jersey) and similar devices are helpful but tend to be too limiting, so, again, cannot be used for sports [15]. The canvas lace-up style brace, Swede-O (North Branch, Minnesota), for example, is less cumbersome, but is less supportive. Other Velcro style straps such as Wrip Wrap (Norco, California) or neoprene sleeves like Pro Orthopaedic (Tuscon, Arizona), provide some support. However, the support provided by these means is no more effective that ordinary ankle taping [15]. Mann [15] proposed a custom thermomold cup with a combination hindfoot brace that has yielded good results despite the need for multiple adjustments before proper fit.

Rehabilitation exercises are an important part of conservative management, and should continue for at least 2 to 3 months [23]. For chronic instability, two consecutive phases of rehabilitation are advocated, namely functional and prophylactic [23]. Initially in the functional phase, all exercises and activities should be pain and symptom free, and be weight bearing and multidirectional [23]. In the prophylactic phase, again, multidirectional movements and strengthening of all muscle groups around the ankle should occur. Emphasis should be put on performing the exercises with the ankle in plantar flexion and inversion, with the joint being progressively stressed to meet the demands imposed on it [23]. There may be a role for ankle taping/bracing in the prophylactic rehabilitation phase, but it is recognized that no type of taping/bracing will prevent all future injuries [23].

Historically, athletes would use ankle taping in an attempt to prevent ankle sprains. Ankle taping is effective in restricting range of motion, and decreases the incidence of ankle sprains [24,25]. However, up to 50% of the stabilizing effect of ankle taping is lost after as only 10 minutes of exercise [26]. Because of this deterioration of support and the cost of tape, removable and reusable ankle braces were designed as an alternative to taping. Overall, braces are effective in preventing, decreasing, or slowing motions that cause lateral ankle ligamentous injuries [27,28], although braces may not to be as effective as freshly applied tape [27]. However, unlike tape, braces offer the advantage of being easily adjusted if and when support becomes compromised. Clinically, braces appear to be at least as effective as tape in the prevention of lateral ankle sprains [29,30]. One study showed that in basketball players the rate of ankle injury was triple that that in nonbraced players [30]. Probably, braces also have a proprioceptive effect in addition to a purely mechanical one.

Regardless of the type of bracing or taping used, a good rehabilitation program will contain an individually designed exercise regime to improve local muscle strength and endurance. Fully activated and strong peroneal muscles are probably the best protection for the near maximally inverted ankle at foot strike [31].

Summary

Chronic ankle instability is a significant cause of morbidity. There are well-documented and effective surgical options for managing this condition. However, conservative management can be a viable option in selected patients. Failure of conservative management can be an indication for surgery if morbidity warrants it. Surgery can be delayed without necessarily affecting outcome.

References

[1] Evans DL. Recurrent instability of the ankle—a method of surgical treatment. Proc R Soc Med 1953;46:343–4.
[2] Keeman JN. Commentaar enkelspecial. Reuma Trauma 1990;1:34–5.
[3] Weber JM, Maleski RM. Clin Podiatr Med Surg 2002;19:309–18.
[4] Stormont D, Morrey B, An K, et al. Stability of the loaded ankle: relationship between articular restraint and primary and secondary static restraints. Am J Sports Med 1985;13: 295–300.
[5] Brostrom L. Sprained ankles: 1. Anatomic lesions in recent sprains. Acta Chir Scand 1964; 128:483–95.
[6] Lynch SA, Renstrom AFH. Treatment of acute lateral ankle ligament rupture in the athlete: conservative versus surgical treatment. Sports Med 1999;27(1):61–71.
[7] Bahr R, Pena F, Shine J, et al. Mechanics of the anterior drawer and talar tilt tests. A cadaveric study of lateral ligament injuries of the ankle. Acta Orthop Scand 1997;68(5):435–41.
[8] Tohyama H, Yasuda K, Ohkoshi Y, et al. Anterior drawer test for acute anterior talofibular ligament injuries of the ankle. How much load should be applied during the test? Am J Sports Med 2003;31(2):226–32.
[9] Saltzman CL, el-Khoury GY. The hindfoot alignment view. Foot Ankle Int 1995;16(9): 572–6.

[10] Karlsson J, Lansinger O, Faxen E. Lateral instability of the ankle joint (2). Active training programs can prevent surgery. Lakartidningen 1991;88(15):1404–7.

[11] Frost SC, Amendola A. Is stress radiography necessary in the diagnosis of acute or chronic ankle instability? Clin J Sport Med 1999;9(1):40–5.

[12] Karlsson J, Lansinger O. Chronic lateral instability of the ankle in athletes. Sports Med 1993; 16(5):355–65.

[13] Trevino SG, Davis P, Hecht PJ. Management of acute and chronic lateral ligament injuries of the ankle. Orthop Clin North Am 1994;25(1):1–16.

[14] Karlsson J, Lansinger O. Lateral instability of the ankle joint (1). Non-surgical treatment is the first choice—20 per cent may need ligament surgery. Lakartidningen 1991;88(15): 1399–402.

[15] Mann RA. Athletic injuries to the soft tissues of the foot and ankle. In: Mann RA, Coughlin MJ, editors. Surgery of the foot and ankle. 7th edition. St Louis (MO): Mosby; 1999. p. 1153–65.

[16] Drez D, Young J, Waldman D. Non operative treatment of double lateral ligament tears of the ankle. Am J Sports Med 1982;10:197–200.

[17] Smith RW, Reischl SF. Treatment of ankle sprains in young athletes. Am J Sports Med 1986; 14:465–71.

[18] Clanton TO. Instability of the subtalar joint. Orthop Clin North Am 1989;20:583–92.

[19] Karlsson J, Andreasson G. The effect of external ankle support in chronic lateral ankle joint instability. Am J Sports Med 1992;20:257–61.

[20] Gauffin H, Tropp H, Odenrick P. Effect of ankle disk training on postural control in patients with functional instability of the ankle. Int J Sports Med 1988;9:141–4.

[21] Cooper PS. Proprioception in injury prevention and rehabilitation of ankle sprains. In: Sammarco GJ, editor. Rehabilitation of the foot and ankle. St. Louis (MO): Mosby-Year Book; 1995. p. 95–105.

[22] Keefe DT, Haddad SL. Subtalar instability. Etiology, diagnosis and management. Foot Ankle Clin North Am 2002;7:577–609.

[23] Safran MR, Zachazewski JE, Benedetti R, et al. Lateral ankle sprains: a comprehensive review Part 2: treatment and rehabilitation with an emphasis on the athlete. Med Sci Sports Exerc 1999;31(7):S438–47.

[24] Abdenour TE, Saville WA, White RC, et al. The effect of ankle taping upon torque and range of motion. Athl Training 1979;14:227–8.

[25] Delacerde FG. Effect of underwrap conditions on the supportive effectiveness of ankle strapping with tape. J Sports Med 1978;18:77–81.

[26] Fumich RM, Ellison AE, Guerin GJ. The measured effect of taping on combined foot and ankle motion before and after exercise. Am J Sports Med 1981;9:165–70.

[27] Shapiro MS, Kabo JM, Mitchell PW, et al. Ankle sprain prophylaxis: an analysis of the stabilizing effects of braces and tapes. Am J Sports Med 1994;22:78–82.

[28] Siegler S, Liu W, Sennett B, et al. The three dimensional passive support characteristics of ankle braces. J Orthop Sports Phys Ther 1997;26:299–309.

[29] Sharpe SS, Knapik J, Jones B. Ankle braces effectively reduce recurrence of ankle sprains in female soccer players. J Athl Train 1997;32:21–4.

[30] Sitler M, Ryan J, Wheeler B. The efficacy of a semi-rigid ankle stabilizer to reduce acute ankle injuries in basketball: a randomized clinical study at West Point. Am J Sports Med 1994;22: 454–61.

[31] Ashton-Miller JA, Ottaviani RA, Hutchinson C, et al. What best protects the inverted weight-bearing ankle against further inversion? Everter muscle strength compares favorably with shoe height, athletic tape, and three orthoses. Am J Sports Med 1996;24:800–9.

ELSEVIER
SAUNDERS

Foot Ankle Clin N Am
11 (2006) 539–545

FOOT AND
ANKLE CLINICS

Anatomic Repair for Chronic Lateral Ankle Instability

Adam Ajis, BMedSc (Hons Physiol), MBChB, MRCSEd[a],
Alastair S.E. Younger, MB ChB, ChM, MSc, FRCSC[b],
Nicola Maffulli, MD, MS, PhD, FRCS (Orth)[a],*

[a]*Department of Trauma and Orthopaedic Surgery, Keele University School of Medicine,
Thornburrow Drive, Hartshill, Stoke on Trent ST4 7QB Staffs, United Kingdom*
[b]*British Columbia's Foot and Ankle Clinic, Suite 560 1144 Burrard Street, Vancouver,
British Columbia, Canada V6Z 3E8*

Ankle sprains are one of the most common musculoskeletal injuries, accounting for as much as 40% of all athletic injuries [1]. In a recent study, the overall incidence of sprains in its general population was 7 per 1000 person-years [2]. Most of these injuries are lateral ligament sprains from forced inversion with the ankle joint in plantar flexion. In the acute situation, rest, ice, compression, and elevation is the standard accepted management and surgery is rarely indicated. This is then followed by rehabilitation. Early controlled motion and functional bracing has better results than primary surgical repair or casting in the acute setting [3].

Most patients managed conservatively will do well, but up to 20% will have symptoms of functional ankle instability [4]. They will experience recurrent inversion sprains, pain, and difficulty on walking on uneven ground. Supervised rehabilitation aimed at improving ankle proprioception and peroneal muscle strengthening is the mainstay of management. Bracing can be effective in improving symptoms, thereby reducing the need for surgical management.

Patients who continue to sustain multiple recurrent inversion sprains and suffer from chronic ankle instability despite a program of rehabilitation are candidates for surgery. Many different procedures have been described to repair the lateral ankle ligaments and restore stability, with different effects

* Corresponding author.
E-mail address: n.maffulli@keele.ac.uk (N. Maffulli).

1083-7515/06/$ - see front matter © 2006 Elsevier Inc. All rights reserved.
doi:10.1016/j.fcl.2006.07.005

foot.theclinics.com

on ankle and subtalar joint mechanics. Most reconstructive procedures involve either direct late repair of the ligaments or indirect stabilization with the use of tendon grafts. Although most of these reconstructions are effective, the surgeon should choose the simplest method that restores normal ankle anatomy and biomechanics.

Anatomy

In neutral position, the tight fit of the talus between the tibia and fibula stabilizes the ankle joint [5]. The compressive loads imposed under weight bearing enhance osseous stability [5]. With increasing plantar flexion, the osseous constraints are lessened, and the soft tissues are more susceptible to strain and injury [5].

The lateral ankle joint ligamentous complex consists primarily of three structures: the anterior talofibular ligament (ATFL), the calcaneofibular ligament (CFL), and the posterior talofibular ligament (PTFL) (see Fig. 1).

The ATFL is the most anterior structure, and is weakest and most easily injured of these ligaments [6]. The ATFL is often described as a thickening of the lateral joint capsule [7]. When the foot is plantar flexed, the ATFL is vertical, and is the primary stabilizing structure of the ankle during an inversion stress.

The CFL is a round, cord-like extracapsular structure that originates from the inferior distal surface of the fibula, extends posteroinferiorly, deep to the peroneal tendons, and attaches on a small tubercle on the posterior aspect of the lateral calcaneal surface. The CFL is vertical with the foot dorsiflexed, when it becomes the primary ankle stabilizer and secondary subtalar joint stabilizer. Isolated injuries of the CFL are rare.

The PTFL is the strongest and least vulnerable of the three ligaments: isolated ruptures are extremely rare. It is injured in severe ankle sprains after the ATFL and CFL have been disrupted. The PTFL is a trapezoid-shaped structure, which originates from the distal portion of the digital fossa of the

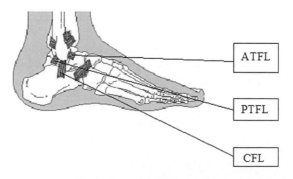

Fig. 1. Lateral ankle ligaments.

fibula and inserts on the posterolateral tubercle of the talus, and on the os trigonum when present.

The Brostrom technique

A curvilinear incision is made over the distal anterior border of the lateral malleolus through skin and subcutaneous tissue. Care is taken to avoid the peroneal tendons inferiorly, the sural nerve (which lies over the peroneal tendons), the lesser saphenous vein, and branches of the superficial peroneal nerve. After dissecting through the subcutaneous tissue, damaged ligaments are identified. The ATFL is a thickening in the anterior capsule (Fig. 2). It is usually torn from the fibula, and the CFL can be identified at the tip of the fibula (Fig. 3).

In the original Brostrom paper, published in 1966, the torn ends of ATFL were shortened and repaired directly with mid-substance suturing [8]. The CFL was not always repaired, and, if it did undergo repair, the same technique was used.

Karlsson and colleagues [9] noted that the ATFL and CFL were usually elongated and scarred rather than disrupted, and recommended shortening the ligaments and reattaching them to the fibula at their anatomic origins via the usage of drill holes. The proximal ligament ends were oversewn to the distal ends to reinforce repair using a Kessler technique (Figs. 4 and 5).

Gould and colleagues [10] described a modification of the Brostrom technique, which included repair of the lateral talocalcaneal ligament and reefing of the lateral ankle retinaculum to the fibula (Fig. 6) in addition to repair of the ATFL and CFL.

Sjolin and colleagues [11] reported the use of periosteal flaps from the distal fibula to help strengthen direct repair. This has the advantage of reinforcing weakened tissues without extensive dissection or morbidity.

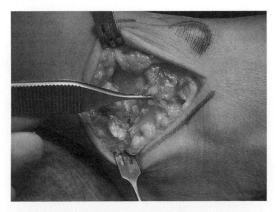

Fig. 2. ATFL demonstrated held by forceps.

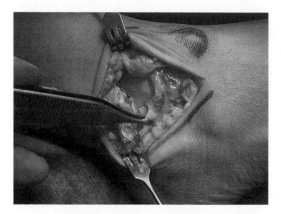

Fig. 3. CFL demonstrated in forceps.

Postoperatively, various different regimes are in use. The authors advocate immobilization of the ankle in plaster for 2 to 3 weeks, with the foot held in eversion and the ankle in neutral dorsiplantar flexion. A removable ankle brace is then fitted and a rehabilitation program is commenced. Passive inversion stretching is avoided for 6 weeks, after which time progressive resistive and proprioceptive exercises are continued for the next 3 months. Between 3 to 6 months, an ankle brace is worn constantly, especially for sports. Most athletes are advised to wear some ankle protection, for example, taping, indefinitely.

Advantages and disadvantages

The Brostrom procedure and its modifications have the advantages of restoration of normal anatomy, preservation of subtalar joint motion, and reduction of morbidity associated with harvesting of tendon grafts as in

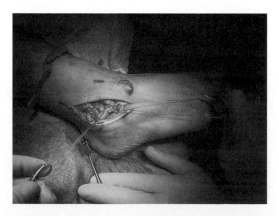

Fig. 4. ATFL ligament ends with Kessler style sutures in place.

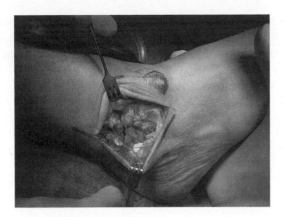

Fig. 5. Sutured ATFL and CFL ligament ends.

the other procedures. The main disadvantage of this technique is inability to adequately stabilize the ankle and/or subtalar joint due to the weakened and scarred tissues used in the repair. Karlsson and colleagues [9] noted that failures in the original Brostrom series tended to occur when the CFL was not reconstructed, perhaps because subtalar motion was not properly controlled.

Results

Brostrom reported successful restoration of functional stability in 51 of 60 patients, 85%, after his late direct repair [8].

Karlsson and colleagues [9] showed with their modification an excellent or good score in 86% of their 152 patients. Analysis of management failures led them to the conclusion that the CFL should always be reconstructed with the ATFL, and that an augmented repair should be considered in

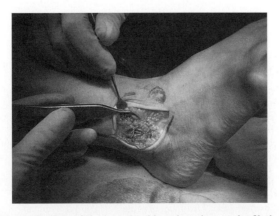

Fig. 6. Reefing of the lateral ankle retinaculum to the fibula.

patients with previous failed direct repairs increased generalized ligamentous laxity and long-standing ankle instability of 10 years or more.

When comparing Brostrom direct repair with more complex tenodesis procedures, in the short to medium term, studies have shown superior results for direct repair [12,13].

Krips and colleagues [14] compared the modified Brostrom technique against the Watson-Jones and Castaing tenodesis procedures with a mean follow-up period in both groups of over 12 years. Tenodesis procedures lead to inferior results in terms of mechanical and functional stability, as well as overall satisfaction in the medium to long term.

Bell and colleagues [15] reported excellent long-term results at 26 years after Brostrom repair using a questionnaire survey.

Summary

Symptomatic ankle instability will develop in up to 20% of patients after inversion injury. Although most patients can be successfully managed with rehabilitation and bracing, some will continue to suffer recurrent ankle instability with activities of daily living, work on uneven terrain, or sports. For this group of patients, we advocate direct anatomic surgical repair with the Brostrom procedure with or without its modifications.

Numerous surgical procedures have been described and shown to be effective, most with an 80% to 90% success rate [1]. Reconstructions using tendon grafts may restrict normal ankle and subtalar joint biomechanics, and have the added risk of more potential complications and morbidity. The Brostrom repair is technically simple, anatomic, and is successful in the short, medium, and longer term. The relative contraindications to this repair are patients with severe ligamentous laxity, excessively weakened defective tissue for direct repair, and patients with previous failed direct repair.

References

[1] Colville MR. Surgical treatment of the unstable ankle. J Am Acad Orthop Surg 1998;6: 368–77.

[2] Holmer P, Sondergaad L, Konradsen L, et al. Epidemiology of sprains in the lateral ankle and foot. Foot Ankle Int 1994;15:72–4.

[3] Kannus P, Renstrom P. Treatment of acute tears of the lateral ligament of the ankle. J Bone Joint Surg Am 1991;73:305–12.

[4] Freeman MAR. Instability of the foot after injuries to the lateral ligament of the ankle. J Bone Joint Surg Br 1965;47:669–77.

[5] Stormont D, Morrey B, An K, et al. Stability of the loaded ankle: relationship between articular restraint and primary and secondary static restraints. Am J Sports Med 1985;13: 295–300.

[6] Brostrom L. Sprained ankles: 1. Anatomic lesions in recent sprains. Acta Chir Scand 1964; 128:483–95.

[7] Lynch SA, Renstrom AFH. Treatment of acute lateral ankle ligament rupture in the athlete: conservative versus surgical treatment. Sports Med 1999;27(1):61–71.

[8] Brostrom L. Sprained ankles VI. Surgical treatment of "chronic" ligament ruptures. Acta Chir Scand 1966;132:551–65.

[9] Karlsson J, Bergsten T, Lansinger O, et al. Reconstruction of the lateral ligaments of the ankle for chronic lateral instability. J Bone Joint Surg Am 1998;70:581–8.

[10] Gould N, Seligson D, Gassman J. Early and late repair of lateral ligaments of the ankle. Foot Ankle 1980;1:84–9.

[11] Sjolin SU, Dons-Jensen H, Simonsen O. Reinforced anatomical reconstruction of the anterior talofibular ligament in chronic anterolateral instability using a periosteal flap. Foot Ankle 1991;12:15–8.

[12] Hennrikus WL, Mapes RC, Lyons PM, et al. Outcomes of the Chrismann-Snook and modified Brostrom procedures for chronic lateral ankle instability. A prospective, randomised comparison. Am J Sports Med 1996;24:400–4.

[13] Mabit C, Chaudruc JM, Fiorenza F, et al. Lateral ligament reconstruction of the ankle: comparative study of peroneus brevis tenodesis versus periosteal ligamentoplasty. Foot Ankle Surg 1998;4:71–6.

[14] Krips R, van Dijk CN, Halasi T, et al. Long-term outcome of anatomical reconstruction versus tenodesis for the treatment of chronic anterolateral instability of the ankle joint: a multicentre study. Foot Ankle Int 2001;22:415–21.

[15] Bell JS, Mologne TS, Stitler DF, et al. Twenty-six year results after Brostrom procedure for chronic lateral instability. Am J Sports Med 2006;34:975–8.

ELSEVIER
SAUNDERS

Foot Ankle Clin N Am
11 (2006) 547–565

FOOT AND
ANKLE CLINICS

Operative Management of Ankle Instability: Reconstruction with Open and Percutaneous Methods

Norman Espinosa, MD, Jonathan Smerek, MD, Anish R. Kadakia, MD, Mark S. Myerson, MD*

Institute for Foot and Ankle Reconstruction, Mercy Medical Center, 301 St. Paul Street, Baltimore, Maryland 21202, USA

Healthy and functional ankle and subtalar joints provide adaptation of the foot when walking on uneven ground. Congruous bony anatomy and an intact lateral ligamentous complex are the basis for physiologic function. Ligamentous ankle sprains are very common, and may be associated with significant disruption of the supportive structures of the ankle and subtalar joints. Approximately 85% of all ankle sprains involve the lateral structures [1,2]. There is an increasing frequency of lateral ankle sprains in the adolescent and young adult, with males and athletes most commonly affected [3].

Chronic pain after an ankle sprain, recurrent sprains, an ongoing inability to walk on uneven ground, or discomfort with start–stop maneuvers ("giving way") may indicate chronic instability. The prevalence of chronic instability after lateral ankle injury ranges from 10% up to 30% [4–8]. Inadequate management of an acute injury, with poor and insufficient healing of the ankle ligaments, can result in chronic disability. An accurate diagnosis is mandatory to embark on the proper management regimen and to optimize outcomes.

Conservative management using strengthening exercises, proprioceptive training, taping, or stirrup braces may reestablish mechanical stability and enhance proprioceptive input to the peroneal tendon complex [9]. However, it is unlikely that conservative management will yield success in patients who have an active lifestyle or in those whose symptoms interfere with their activities of daily living. When conservative management fails, or when

* Corresponding author.
E-mail address: mark4feet@aol.com (M.S. Myerson).

1083-7515/06/$ - see front matter © 2006 Elsevier Inc. All rights reserved.
doi:10.1016/j.fcl.2006.07.003
foot.theclinics.com

disabling pain and instability persists, reconstruction of the lateral ligaments should be considered [8].

Surgical repair of the lateral ankle ligaments is categorized based on the type of repair, that is, anatomic versus nonanatomic. Adequate reconstruction of ankle stability is always challenging. Obviously, restoration of anatomic and adequate static function of the anterior tibiofibular (ATFL) and the calcaneofibular ligament (CFL) is required to achieve this goal. Once the ligaments are repaired, the results of surgery should be durable and preserve full range of motion at the ankle and subtalar joint [10]. Numerous surgical options for ankle stabilization exist. Many of the described procedures are modifications of well-established, traditional techniques. This review focuses on surgical management of ankle instability by means of the common open approaches, and reports a novel minimally invasive method. Additionally, the history, anatomy, and biomechanics of reconstructive surgery of the lateral ankle ligaments are reviewed.

Historic perspective

Originally, nonanatomic methods of lateral ankle ligament reconstruction were introduced to restore the function of either the CFL or the ATFL. Nilsonne, in 1932, described a nonanatomic autogenous ATFL reconstruction using the peroneus brevis tendon [11]. Elmslie, in 1934, used an autograft transfer of free fascia lata [12]. Although the original method of Nilsonne did not become widespread, the basic concepts of modern ankle ligament reconstruction had been set in motion. Nilsonne described detachment of the peroneus brevis at the level of the musculotendinous junction. Proximally, the muscle of peroneus brevis was sutured to the peroneus longus, and the distal part of the peroneus brevis tendon was placed in a subperiosteal groove through the fibula oriented from posterosuperior to anteroinferior. The tendon of peroneus brevis was then secured in the subperiostal channel. In 1952, Watson-Jones routed the tendon of peroneus brevis through the fibula into the neck of the talus, and then sutured back onto itself [13]. Lee has modified this method since [14].

The use of the peroneus brevis tendon for lateral ankle ligament reconstruction has since become increasingly popular among, and is used most often. Evans modified Nilsonne's technique by placing a drill hole through the fibula to produce a subperiosteal tunnel. The tendon of the peroneus brevis has been fed through the osseous tunnel of the fibula and secured posteroproximally at the superior peroneal retinaculum [15]. Although Evans' modification does not reconstruct the ATFL or the CFL in an anatomic fashion, it is still used today because it is technically easy. Also today, several modifications of the Evans and Watson-Jones techniques exist. Concerns arose regarding optimal resistance against anterior displacement, internal rotation, and adduction because of lack of anatomic reconstruction of the ATFL or CFL. The Watson-Jones and Evans procedures are associated with high rates of persistent subjective instability [16,17]. In addition, approximately 50% of all patients who underwent these reconstructions still have a persistent anterior drawer test [18,19].

In contrast, Chrisman and Snook, in 1969, completely modified the method of Elmslie [20]. Instead of a fascia lata graft, they used the tendon of peroneus brevis as a transfer to reconstruct the ATFL and CFL. Because of its triangular routing, this technique restricted inversion of the ankle and the subtalar joint, and annihilated anterior laxity [21]. Additionally, there was a lower rate of subjective instability when compared with both the Evans and Watson-Jones procedures [22]. Smith and colleagues [23] published a variation of this technique in 1995, and recently, Acevedo and Myerson [24] presented a new modification of the classic Chrisman-Snook technique avoiding drill holes in the talus. However, all these procedures do not reproduce normal ankle kinematics.

In 1966, Broström described a reconstructive procedure that restored the anatomy of the ATFL and CFL using available tissue [25], restoring the normal kinematics of the ankle and subtalar joints. This concept was based on detailed anatomic and clinical observations of sprained ankles. The torn ends of the injured ligament did not atrophy and retract [4,26,27]. Although Haig, in 1950, reported an anatomic repair using local tissue augmentation, Broström's procedure was the first in terms of a primary, direct, and anatomic repair of the lateral ankle region. The procedure requires only a limited surgical exposure, and provides a viable option for many patients with chronic ankle instability. The procedure uses the available scarred or stretched ATFL and CFL, and shortens them by reefing them in vest-over pants fashion. The Broström procedure and its later published variation by Gould [28–31] with additional reefing of the extensor retinaculum have remained standard techniques in the management of ankle instability with good to excellent long-term results.

The last 2 decades have seen a significant improvement in the understanding of the anatomic and biomechanical behavior of the ankle and subtalar joint. More sophisticated operative instruments, allograft soft tissue, and bioabsorbable fixation provide useful platforms to establish new minimal invasive techniques, with similar kinematics and results as more invasive open procedures. One of these techniques is the percutaneous reconstruction by means of a hamstring allograft tendon and interference screws, as originally described by Myerson and colleagues [32].

Ligamentous anatomy of the lateral ankle and subtalar joint

The ankle complex includes three joints: the tibiotalar, subtalar, and the distal tibofibular syndesmosis. These articulations act as a combined osseous and soft tissue (ligaments, capsule, retinacula) support complex, which provides proprioception, stabilization, and control over the movement of the talus and calcaneus around their axes of motion.

When focusing on the lateral ligamentous complex, there are three important structures, namely the ATFL, CFL, and the posterior talofibular ligament (PTFL). Of these, the CFL is the only one that spans both the tibiotalar and talocalcaneal joints. The ATFL originates at the distal anterior fibula, inserts on the body of the talus, and blends into the anterior joint capsule, approximately 18 mm above the subtalar joint line. It is approximately 20 mm long, 8 mm wide, 2 mm thick, and spans the anterior ankle joint. The angle in relation to the floor averages approximately 75° [33–35].

The CFL originates from the anterior border of the distal lateral malleolus, very close to the origin of the ATFL, and attaches to a small tubercle posterior and superior to the peroneal tubercle of the calcaneus, approximately 13 mm distal and posterior to the subtalar joint line. It is confluent with the peroneal tendon sheath. The CFL is 20 to 30 mm long, almost 5 mm wide and 3 to 5 mm thick. Together, the ATFL and CFL form an angle of about 105° in the sagittal plane, and an angle averaging 90° to 100° in the frontal plane, which must be recreated during anatomic surgical reconstruction [33,36–41].

The inferior extensor retinaculum can be used to reinforce ATFL and CFL reconstructions. It is divided into three bands (lateral, intermediate, and medial roots) that retain the extensor digitorum longus, extensor digitorum brevis, and peroneus tertius. The inferior extensor retinaculum is attached to the lateral talus and calcaneus. Together with the CFL, the lateral root of the inferior extensor retinaculum constitutes the superficial ligamentous support of the subtalar joint [42].

The interosseous talocalcaneal ligament, although not a lateral structure, ensures adequate function of the hindfoot, and is the strongest bond between the calcaneus and the talus. It originates at the most medial part of the sinus tarsi with some fibers attach to the deep portion of the deltoid ligament, and courses downward and lateral to the sulcus calcanei, where it blends with the most medial fibers of the cervical ligament. The cervical ligament is located within the sinus tarsi, and runs in an oblique fashion from the neck of the talus to the superior surface of the calcaneus. The sural nerve courses behind and inferior to the lateral malleolus, with an average distance from the tip of 13 mm [43].

Biomechanical aspects

Biomechanics of the normal and unstable ankle and the effect of reconstruction

A stable ankle results from a perfect interplay of static (bones, ligaments, retinaculum) and dynamic anatomic structures (muscles, tendons). The role of bony and ligamentous stabilizers of the ankle and subtalar joints depends on the load and position of the foot and ankle in space. They provide pro-prioception, stabilization, and limitation of nonphysiologic motion about the lateral ankle. The articular surfaces seem to contribute at least some stability in rotation and inversion [44].

Motion at the ankle is multiplanar, and linked to the tibia [45]. The course of movement within the ankle joint is predominantly from plantar-flexion to dorsiflexion, but has minimal components of internal and external rotation. In contrast, the subtalar joint follows more complex kinematics. The calcaneus rotates around the interosseus ligament, resulting in a screw-like motion associated with translation and rotation. Motion at the subtalar joint is triplanar, with inversion (calcaneus turns inward) and eversion (calcaneus turns outward) [46,47].

Ankle motion is highly dependant on the supporting ligamentous lateral structures. In plantarflexion, the ATFL becomes taut and the CFL remains loose. The ATFL primarily restricts internal rotation of the talus in the mor-tise [48]. The ATFL exhibits the highest degree of deformation, that is, greatest strain, but the lowest load to failure when compared with the CFL [49,50]. The relative strength of the CFL is approximately three times greater than that for the ATFL [49,51]. The CFL stabilizes the subtalar joint, inhibits adduction, and exerts its greatest effect in the neutral and dorsiflexed position. In dorsiflexion, the CFL approaches a vertical position with respect to the subtalar joint, and acts as a true collateral ligament, pre-venting talar tilting. With sectioning of the CFL, the rotation of the subtalar joint was increased by 20%, and adduction of the subtalar joint by 61% to 77% [52]. The combined function of the ATFL and CFL prevents talar tilt. Sectioning either the ATFL or CFL alone did not result in talar tilt, but sec-tioning both ligaments leads to an average talar tilt of 21° [53]. Also, external rotation of the leg occurred with inversion averaging 11° in intact specimens. Interestingly, this external rotation increased with further sectioning of the ATFL and CFL [53]. Other authors have demonstrated that the anterolateral joint capsule adds mechanical stability to the ankle [54]. Inversion is accompanied by a mandatory external rotation of the leg. In the intact hind foot, this rotation takes place at the subtalar joint. In the injured ankle joint without stabilizing ligaments, this rotation takes place at the tibiotalar joint [34,55]. Given these data, ankle instability could be a form of axial rotational instability alone. As most ankle sprains occur in an adducted, plantarflexed, and inverted position, the ATFL is most prone to injury. The second most common combination is rupture of both the ATFL and CFL. An isolated CFL tear is rare.

Each technique of lateral ligament reconstruction alters the normal kinematics of ankle motion. Nonanatomic repairs, such as the Watson-Jones, Evans, and Chrisman-Snook techniques, all restrict motion at both the ankle and subtalar joints. This effect is far more pronounced in these procedures than in an anatomic repair. Anatomic repairs are biomechanically more favorable than any nonanatomic variant. For example, the Watson-Jones procedure resulted in more restricted ankle motion than the Brostrom repair [56]. Also, the Brostrom repair restored more closely the normal ligament force patterns. Hollis and colleagues [16], studying the effect of the Evans, Watson-Jones and Chrisman-Snook procedures, showed decreased laxity after all reconstruction techniques during pronation and supination. The Evans and Chrisman-Snook techniques produced greater mechanical stability during anterior–posterior loading than the Watson-Jones method. Although the Brostrom procedure primarily stabilizes the ankle, the nonanatomic reconstructive techniques can limit motion at the subtalar joint [57]. Anecdotally, the addition of the Gould modification of the Brostrom procedure also tightens up the subtalar joint due to the extension of the extensor retinaculum into the sinus tarsi. Nonanatomic procedures also permit some increased motion when compared with ankles with normal ligament configuration.

Liu and Baker confirmed the effectiveness of the Brostrom procedure in terms of mechanical restraint. They showed that the Chrisman-Snook, Watson-Jones, and Brostrom techniques reduced anterior drawer and talar tilt, but with a far better result for the latter technique [58].

Preoperative workup

History and physical examination

A systematic and complete history and examination is the key to understanding the patterns and contributing factors of instability. In addition, it ensures proper selection of the correct surgical procedure. Freeman and colleagues [5,59] defined the term functional instability to describe the subjective complaint of the ankle "giving way," which he attributed to proprioceptive defects. Mechanical instability results from anatomic factors altering the normal kinematics of at least one joint at the ankle. When describing ankle sprains, the terms ankle ligament laxity, lateral ankle instability, and chronic ankle instability are often used interchangeably. Laxity is a physical sign objectively detected on examination, such as a positive anterior drawer or increased inversion, and is synonimous of mechanical instability. Lateral ankle instability is the presence of an unstable ankle due to lateral ligamentous injury. The patient may describe this as the ankle giving way. Chronic ankle instability refers to repetitive episodes of instability resulting in recurrent ankle sprains, and is synonimous of functional instability. It should be noted that laxity and instability are not interchangeable terms, and that the degree of mechanical instability and functional instability is not necessarily correlated.

The exact location of pain and the circumstances that give rise to the pain should be carefully noted. Pain does not normally accompany ankle instability. Pain can either be deep in the ankle, and invariably associated with an osteochondral defect, or superficial, in which case a tear of the peroneal tendon is often present. There are also patients with chronic ankle instability who have experienced acute injury to the hindfoot with fractures of the anterior process of the calcaneus, and the lateral process of the talus, which may not have been diagnosed. Patients with chronic instability often complain of recurrent sprains, inability to walk on uneven terrain, and report symptoms associated with impingement within the medial and lateral gutters. It is important to ascertain whether the symptoms are present when the patient walks on a flat surface, or whether they only occur when the patient walks on uneven ground. If complaints of instability are present on flat ground surfaces, the assumption is that the instability is more severe, and possibly associated with hindfoot deformity, including heel varus. At times there is associated hypertrophy and inflammation of the peroneal tendons, and rupture of the tendon longus or brevis after repetitive ankle sprains [60]. Any history of prior injury or surgery of the ankle and neurologic disorder (Charcot-Marie-Tooth) must be noted. Patients with pes cavovarus or subtle heel varus are at greater risk for lateral ankle instability [61,62]. Finally, one should assess the activity level and physical demands of the patient, because this is a most important determinant in the choice of surgery.

A thorough clinical examination should test all structures of the ankle. Particular attention should be paid to any alteration of the hindfoot, especially varus malalignment (Fig. 1), hyperlaxity (Fig. 2), and tarsal coalition. Tenderness on palpation over the ATFL and CFL may indicate injury. The longer the time interval between injury and examination, the lower the specificity of tenderness. The peroneal tendons and sinus tarsi should be thoroughly examined. In patients with recurrent ankle instability, the peroneal tendons are usually weak, and require preoperative strengthening and retraining. Swelling and tenderness over the peroneal sheath can indicate possible longitudinal tear of the tendons. The range of motion at the ankle should be noted, together

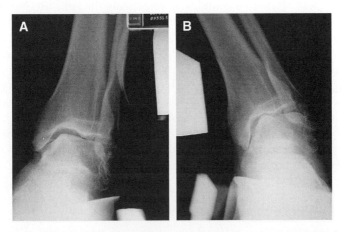

Fig. 1. A patient with varus hindfoot malalignment (*A*). On stress testing, the patient showed a clear pathological laxity of the ankle joint with marked talar tilt (*B*).

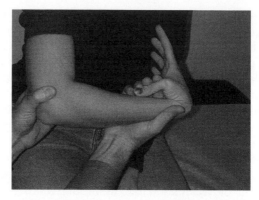

Fig. 2. A patient with chronic ankle instability and marked generalized joint hyperlaxity.

with the presence of anterior or posterior impingement. Laxity of the ATFL is tested using the anterior drawer test [63–65]. ATFL and CFL laxity are also tested by talar tilt manipulations, which is best evaluated by stress fluoroscopic or radiograph examination. It should however the noted.

Imaging

Plain weight-bearing radiographs may reveal bony lesions. Stress radiographs can be performed in attempt to assess mechanical integrity of the ligaments. Often plain radiographs are noncontributory, and the use and reliability of stress radiographs is still debated [66–69]. Two methods of stress radiographs are commonly used: the anterior drawer test and the talar tilt test [70,71]. The former test assesses the integrity of the ATFL [65]. Normal values for anterior displacement range between 2.5 and 3 mm. An anterior displacement greater than 6 mm is considered frankly pathologic. The CFL is tested by applying a varus stress to the ankle and measuring the talar tilt. Normal talar tilt values range from 10° to 23°. Some authors recommend using the differences in talar tilt between the normal and pathologic ankle, with a side to side difference of 9° being clinically significant [72]. Talar tilt exceeding 15° may indicate a high probability of a complete CFL tear. However, as the management of chronic ankle instability is based on the functional deficit that they determine, and does not depend on the degree of ankle instability on stress views, stress radiographs may well have little clinical relevance.

The use of a CT or MRI scanning is reserved to selected patients on the basis of additional conditions (ie, anterior capsular impingement or osteochondral defect) present.

Selection of surgery

A surgeon's personal experience and philosophy of management determine what procedure shall be selected to manage ankle instability in a given patient. In addition to the findings on clinical examination and imaging, the physical demands and lifestyle of a patient contribute heavily to the decision-making process. Once the decision to pursue surgical reconstruction has been reached, two questions need to be answered: Should the approach be open or percutaneous, and should it proceed in a nonanatomic or anatomic manner. Finally, regardless of the procedure selected, one must determine the need for additional surgery, including calcaneus osteotomy, peroneal tendon repair, or ankle arthroscopy.

Open or percutaneous approach?

We perform an anatomic percutaneous reconstruction wherever possible. This procedure is particularly indicated in the absence of deformity and pain. If the ankle pain is either caused by an anterior capsular impingement syndrome or a cartilage lesion, an arthroscopy may be performed simultaneously, and this percutaneous approach then has great advantages. One of the problems with any open procedure following ankle arthroscopy is the disruption of soft tissue planes as a result of extravasation of fluid into the subcutaneous and interstitial tissues. The percutaneous approach then avoids the necessary dissection associated with open surgery. Clearly, if deformity is present and an osteotomy of the calcaneus is to be performed, then, in addition to the lateral incision over the heel, a short puncture can be made anteriorly over the ankle for insertion of the graft, avoiding a longer incision. If peroneal tendon pathology is suspected, then a short incision is made over the peroneal tendons, the sheath opened, and following tendon repair a decision can be made regarding the type of ankle reconstruction. If a split of the peroneus brevis is not reparable, then the anterior half of the peroneus brevis can be used for a nonanatomic reconstruction using a modified Chrisman-Snook procedure. If the peroneal tendon cannot be used for the ankle reconstruction, then an anatomic procedure can be performed with a hamstring allograft as described below. The real advantage of an open approach lies in facilitated access to tendon and intraarticular pathology, but, as noted here, this does not imply an extensile incision.

Anatomic or nonanatomic reconstruction?

Once the decision has been made to either perform an open or percutaneous repair, the type of reconstruction must be chosen. A surgeon can choose between anatomic reconstructions such as the Broström-Gould or the percutaneous hamstring allograft procedures, or nonanatomic techniques, including the modified Elmslie, Chrisman-Snook, or the combined Broström-Evans procedures [20,73,74]. Frequently, surgeons select a procedure with which they are comfortable. This should nonetheless be performed within certain guidelines, paying attention to generalized ligamentous laxity, heavy demand on the ankle, the athlete, and the need to control the subtalar and the ankle joints.

The high-performance athlete

As a generalization, one should try not to sacrifice either the peroneal or the hamstring tendons in an athlete. Furthermore, one should avoid any procedure that tightens up the subtalar joint, thereby eliminating many of the nonanatomic procedures. Perhaps the epitomy of this type of athlete is the gymnast or the ballet dancer, for whom a perfect range of motion without any tightness of the subtalar joint is desirable. In most, if not all, athletes, preservation of strong eversion is essential, and the peroneal tendons should not be used to perform the reconstruction. As with the peroneals, there is no reason to sacrifice the hamstrings in the athlete to perform a hamstring autograft reconstruction. Although a hamstring autograft reconstruction has been described, this should be avoided in runners or in those athletes who are involved in "stop-and-go" sports [75]. The sacrifice of a hamstring may compromise terminal flexion torque, which is highly detrimental to the sprinting athlete. The question then arises when to perform a Brostrom or a percutaneous hamstring allograft procedure. In general, any procedure that facilitates recovery, enables a rapid return to sporting activity, and has a minimum rate of complications is desirable, and for many of these patients should be the management of choice. Although nonanatomic, the technique avoids disruption of the peroneal tendons and preserves mobility of the ankle joint. Conversely, in the heavy-weight athlete (boxer, football lineman, wrestler, or body builder), or in those individuals with heel varus, increased stiffness at the ankle is desired. This is achieved by employing a modification of the Elmslie or Chrisman-Snook technique. Some authors use a combined Brostrom-Evans method, which incorporates nonanatomic and anatomic aspects of lateral ankle reconstruction [74].

The "low-demand" patient with an unstable ankle

The Broström-Gould augmentation is anatomic, and yields durable good to excellent outcomes, even in the long term [29]. It is relatively easy to perform, and is appropriate for most patients presenting with ankle instability. It should be used with caution in patients with hyperlaxity, or those with prior failed stabilization surgery, or in patients suffering from work-related injury [76]. These conditions are better managed by a nonanatomic procedure that stiffens the ankle.

To address the resultant ankle stiffness of nonanatomic procedures, a new percutaneous hamstring allograft method with biointerference screws has been developed [32]. Although nonanatomic, it does not sacrifice the peroneal tendons, and allows better control to avoid joint stiffness. Whenever possible, this procedure is used for ankle ligament reconstruction. If there is no available allograft tissue, an Elmslie, modified Chrisman-Snook, or split Evans procedure can be performed. Patients with cavovarus may require a calcaneal osteotomy or a first metatarsal dorsiflexion osteotomy.

Surgical techniques

The modified Broström-Gould procedure

If one chooses to manage a patient with an unstable ankle with the Broström procedure (Fig. 3), the choice of incision is critical . One can follow either the traditional hockey stick or J-type incision. If there are any concerns regarding the integrity of the peroneal tendons, an alternative longitudinal incision toward the posterior margin of the fibula should be used. This provides simultaneous inspection of the peroneal tendons and repair of the CFL. An open cheilectomy of the anterior tibiotalar osteophytes from these approaches is easily performed if indicated. The superficial peroneal nerve is in danger at the distal end of the incision, and must be protected.

Dissection should proceed meticulously to identify all retinacular structures. After subcutaneous dissection, the extensor retinaculum is exposed and detached at its inferior insertion in the talar neck, just anterior to the subtalar joint. Although the reconstruction normally proceeds with a pants-over-vest repair of the ATFL, this is often not possible. It is often easier to detach the ATFL at its insertion on the fibula and lift off the remnants of the ATFL from the fibula with a small cuff of periosteum attached. Once the ATFL is advanced and secured, this "flap" is sutured over it. The ATFL can be anchored either by suture anchors or bone tunnels. The latter technique is accomplished by using Kirschner wires to drill holes into the fibula that serve as tunnels for the sutures. The same principles apply for the repair of the CFL, which is exposed after retraction of the peroneal tendons. The ATFL is reconstructed first, with the foot held in neutral dorsiflexion and slight eversion. Upon closing, the extensor retinaculum can be advanced into the fibula and sutured to the periosteal-ligamentous flap created during reconstruction of ATFL.

The modified Chrisman-Snook procedure

In 2000, Acevedo and Myerson presented a modification of the original Chrisman-Snook procedure (Fig. 4) [24]. The modification does not require a talar drill hole, and uses a through and through calcaneal tunnel. The advantage of this modification is that it can be used in the presence of a severe rupture of the peroneus brevis tendon, when the split peroneus brevis portion can be used for reconstruction.

The incision proceeds by paralleling the peroneal tendons. It should not extend more than 6 cm proximal to the tip of the fibula. The length of the rerouted tendon strip is usually about 8 cm. In such instances, the tendon is sufficiently strong to serve as the reconstruction. To avoid further splitting the peroneal brevis tendon distally, a stay suture can be placed in the split.

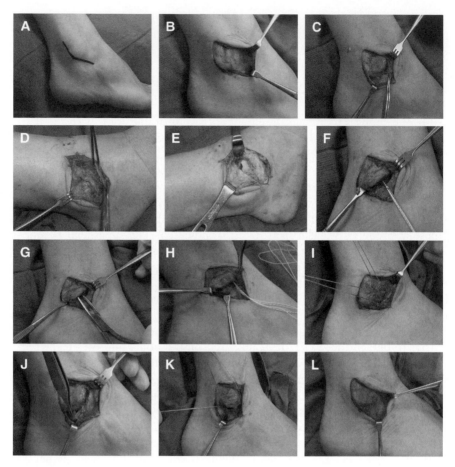

Fig. 3. After having done the incision in either the traditional hockey stick or J-type fashion (*A*), the subcutaneous dissection is started and the extensor retinaculum is exposed (*B*) and detached at its inferior insertion in the talar neck (*C*), just anterior to the subtalar joint. At this point the whole subtalar as well as ankle joint can be inspected (*D*). Please note the osteochondral defect in the talus (*E*). The ATFL can be anchored either by suture anchors or bone tunnels (*F*). This step of the technique is accomplished by using K-wires to drill holes into the fibula that serve as tunnels for the sutures. To achieve better healing of the advanced flap a footprint is created by means of a rongeur (*G*). Normally, the technique uses a pants-over-vest repair of the ATFL, but this is often not possible, so it is easier to detach the ATFL at its insertion on the fibula and lift off the remnants of the ATFL from the fibula with a small cuff of periosteum attached (*H*). Once the ATFL is advanced and secured, this "flap" is sutured over it (*I*). The same principles apply for the repair of the CFL (*J–L*).

A 4.5-mm drill hole is produced, starting at the anterior aspect of the tip of the fibula, running through the body of the fibula, and exiting the posterior cortex. The drill should exit anterior to the peroneal tendon sheath. The tendon is passed anterior to posterior in the bony tunnel. Care should be taken to pass the tendon graft lateral to the peroneus longus tendon to provide stability

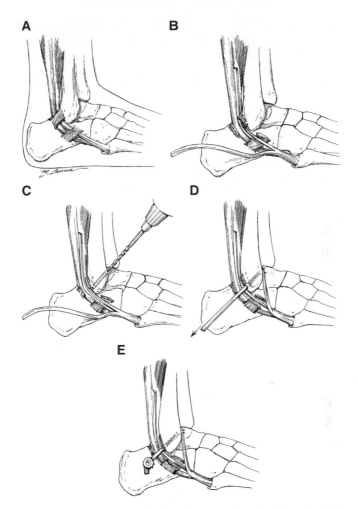

Fig. 4. A 6- to 10-cm long incision parallel to the peroneal tendons is made. The length of the rerouted tendon strip is usually about 8 cm (*A*). To avoid further splitting the peroneal brevis tendon distally, a stay suture can be placed in the split (*B*). A 4.5-mm drill hole is produced starting at the anterior aspect of the tip of the fibula, running through the body of the fibula, and exiting the posterior cortex. The drill should exit anterior to the peroneal tendon sheath (*C*). The tendon is passed anterior to posterior in the bony tunnel (*D*). Care should be taken to pass the tendon graft lateral to the peroneus longus tendon to provide stability and prevent subluxation of the peroneal longus and the remaining peroneus brevis. A drill hole is made at the origin of the CFL on the calcaneus and directed toward the sustentaculum tali. The graft is then passed from lateral to medial. Once the tension is optimal, a biointerference or titanium screw with a washer can be inserted from lateral to medial to fix the tendon in the calcaneus (*E*).

and prevent subluxation of the peroneal longus and the remaining peroneal brevis. Next, a drill hole is begun at the origin of the CFL on the calcaneus and directed toward the sustentaculum. The drill exits the medial border of the calcaneus, a small incision is made medially, and the neurovascular structures are protected. The tip of a suction drain is placed over the tip of the drill and pushed through the calcaneus from medial to lateral. The graft is then passed from lateral to medial. The ankle is positioned in dorsiflexion and eversion with maximal tension on the graft. Once the tension is optimal, a biointerference or titanium screw with a washer can be inserted from lateral to medial to fix the tendon in the calcaneus.

Percutaneous hamstring allograft reconstruction

The key to the percutaneous approach is a thorough understanding of surface anatomy and the liberal use of adjuvant fluoroscopy. A hamstring allograft is prepared (Fig. 5) and trimmed to a thickness of 4 mm, with Krackow-type whip stitches on either end. The entire length of the graft may be used, but the length may be approximated by laying the graft on the skin and simulating the course of the tendon. The graft is kept irrigated in saline/antibiotic solution. The lateral aspect of the neck of the talus is visualized under fluoroscopy, and marked with a guide pin for a 5.0-mm bioabsorbable screw. The guide wire is inserted perpendicular to the talus, midway between the superior and inferior borders of the lateral wall. A 5.5-mm drill is inserted to a depth of 17 mm in the talus. Subsequently, a talus blind tunnel technique is used [31]. A 5.0-mm bioabsorbable screw is inserted with the tendon for an interference fit.

A guide wire for a 4.5-mm drill is then passed percutaneously through the distal fibula, from anterior to posterior, starting 1 cm proximal from the distal tip. A 5-mm incision is made both at the anterior and posterior extents of the guide wire to facilitate passing of the graft. A cannulated 4.5-mm drill produces the fibular tunnel. The tunnel should pass just anterior to the peroneal tendon sheath. The graft is then passed from the talar neck incision, staying on the lateral bony surface of the talus, and then from anterior to posterior in the fibula tunnel. A final 5-mm incision is made over the lateral calcaneal wall, just inferior to the CFL insertion, inferior to the peroneal tendons, and dorsal to the sural nerve. The graft is then passed from the posterior fibular incision, superficial to the peroneal tendons, and deep to the sural nerve. A through and through 4.5-mm tunnel is produced in the calcaneus. The graft suture is passed from lateral to medial, and the graft is tensioned with ankle dorsiflexed and the subtalar joint in a neutral postion. A 7.0-mm interference screw is then inserted from lateral to medial to complete the procedure. Stay sutures may be inserted at the anterior insertion to the fibular tunnel if greater stability is required. Weight bearing can commence at 2 weeks, with the start of range of motion exercises and rehabilitation.

Outcomes

The results of surgical intervention for ankle instability are uniformly excellent. In a prospective, randomized study, Hennrikus and colleagues

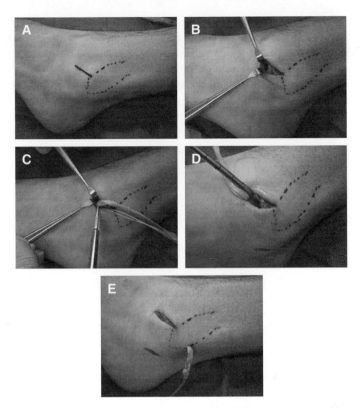

Fig. 5. The lateral aspect of the neck of the talus is visualized by fluoroscopy, and is marked with a guide pin for a 5.0-mm bioabsorbable screw. The guide wire is inserted perpendicular to the talus, midway between the superior and inferior borders of the lateral wall. A 5.5-mm drill hole is made to a final depth of about 17 mm into the talus. Subsequently, a talus blind tunnel technique is used. A 5.0-mm bioabsorbable screw is inserted together with the tendon for an interference fit and to secure the tendon (*A* and *B*). A guide wire for a 4.5-mm drill is then passed percutaneously through the distal fibula, from anterior to posterior, starting 1 cm proximal from the distal tip. A 5-mm incision is made both at the anterior and posterior ends of the guide wire to facilitate passing of the graft. A cannulated 4.5-mm drill is used to produce a fibular tunnel. The tunnel should pass just anterior to the peroneal tendon sheath. The graft is then passed from the talar neck incision (*C* and *D*). Finally, a 5-mm incision is made over the lateral aspect of the calcaneus, inferior to the CFL insertion, inferior to the peroneal tendons, and dorsal to the sural nerve. The graft is passed from the posterior fibular incision, superficial to the peroneal tendons and deep to the sural nerve. A through and through 4.5-mm tunnel is produced in the calcaneus. The graft suture is passed from lateral to medial, and the graft is tensioned with ankle dorsiflexed and the subtalar joint in neutral (*E*).

[77] reported on the outcomes of the Chrisman-Snook and modified Brosström procedures in patients with chronic lateral ankle instability. Regardless of the procedure chosen, both procedures resulted in good to excellent outcomes in more than 80% all ankles. There were significantly more complications in the Chrisman-Snook group, and the modified Broström procedure resulted in higher Sefton scores. Karlsson and colleagues [78]

reported a 87% good or excellent rate in 152 ankles after the Broström procedure. A more recent study investigating the long-term outcome of the modified Broström procedure by Gould showed excellent results of more than 90 points on a scale of possible 100 points [29]. Hamilton and colleagues [79] showed excellent results after the modified Broström procedure in 26 of 28 patients. In contrast, Snook presented the long-term results after Chrisman-Snook procedure with good to excellent results in 93% of the patients. However, in all these studies different scores were used, which makes comparison of the results difficult.

Complications

Despite excellent functional outcomes, complications following reconstructive procedures for lateral ankle instability are fairly common. In the study by Hennrikus and colleagues [77], 25% of patients with a modified Chrisman-Snook procedure had a wound infection, approximately 30% reported tightness at their ankles, and 50% had sensory loss over the distribution of the sural nerve. In 30% of these patients, sensation returned after a period of 12 weeks. In contrast, no wound complications were found in the Broström group. Five percent of patients reported temporary paresthesia, but no permanent nerve injuries occurred. Snook reported a total of 7% permanent sural nerve injuries and a 4% incidence of wound complications. The higher complication rate in the Hennrikus and colleagues [77] study could be attributed to the fact that orthopedic residents under staff supervision had performed most of the surgeries. Additionally, the larger incision puts this anatomic region at a higher risk for colonization with microorganisms.

Summary

Chronic ankle instability affects a large number of young patients. A thorough history and clinical examination are key to proper patient selection. Once the patient decides to undergo operative intervention, the appropriate procedure should be selected according to their physical and lifestyle demands. The surgeon should gain familiarity with the full range of procedures, from open to percutaneous, and anatomic to nonanatomic. With proper patient selection, functional outcomes are excellent, with success rates from 80% to 90%.

References

[1] Liu SH, Nguyen TM. Ankle sprains and other soft tissue injuries. Curr Opin Rheumatol 1999;11:132–7.
[2] Liu SH, Jason WJ. Lateral ankle sprains and instability problems. Clin Sports Med 1994;13: 793–809.

[3] Peters JW, Trevino SG, Renstrom PA. Chronic lateral ankle instability. Foot Ankle 1991;12: 182–91.

[4] Brostrom L, Sundelin P. Sprained ankles. IV. Histologic changes in recent and "chronic" ligament ruptures. Acta Chir Scand 1966;132:248–53.

[5] Freeman MA. Instability of the foot after injuries to the lateral ligament of the ankle. J Bone Joint Surg Br 1965;47:669–77.

[6] Baker JM, Ouzounian TJ. Complex ankle instability. Foot Ankle Clin 2000;5:887–96.

[7] Safran MR, Benedetti RS, Bartolozzi AR 3rd, et al. Lateral ankle sprains: a comprehensive review: part 1: etiology, pathoanatomy, histopathogenesis, and diagnosis. Med Sci Sports Exerc 1999;31:S429–37.

[8] Karlsson J. Ligament injuries of the ankle–what happens later? Non-surgical treatment is effective in 80–90 per cent of cases. Lakartidningen 1998;95:4376–8.

[9] Lofvenberg R, Karrholm J, Lund B. The outcome of nonoperated patients with chronic lateral instability of the ankle: a 20-year follow-up study. Foot Ankle Int 1994;15:165–9.

[10] Baumhauer JF, O'Brien T. Surgical considerations in the treatment of ankle instability. J Athl Train 2002;37:458–62.

[11] Nilsonne R. J Bone Joint Surg Am 1931;14:380.

[12] Elmslie R. Recurrent subluxation of the ankle joint. Proc R Soc Med 1934;37:364–7.

[13] Watson-Jones R. Recurrent forward dislocation of the ankle joint. J Bone Joint Surg Br 1952;134:519.

[14] Lee H. Surgical repair in recurrent dislocation of the ankle joint. J Bone Joint Surg Am 1957; 39:828.

[15] Evans DL. Recurrent instability of the ankle; a method of surgical treatment. Proc R Soc Med 1953;46:343–4.

[16] Hollis JM, Blasier RD, Flahiff CM, et al. Biomechanical comparison of reconstruction techniques in simulated lateral ankle ligament injury. Am J Sports Med 1995;23:678–82.

[17] Younes C, Fowles JV, Fallaha M, et al. Long-term results of surgical reconstruction for chronic lateral instability of the ankle: comparison of Watson-Jones and Evans techniques. J Trauma 1988;28:1330–4.

[18] van der Rijt AJ, Evans GA. The long-term results of Watson-Jones tenodesis. J Bone Joint Surg Br 1984;66:371–5.

[19] Orava S, Jaroma H, Weitz H, et al. Radiographic instability of the ankle joint after Evans' repair. Acta Orthop Scand 1983;54:734–8.

[20] Chrisman OD, Snook GA. Reconstruction of lateral ligament tears of the ankle. An experimental study and clinical evaluation of seven patients treated by a new modification of the Elmslie procedure. J Bone Joint Surg Am 1969;51:904–12.

[21] Colville MR, Marder RA, Zarins B. Reconstruction of the lateral ankle ligaments. A biomechanical analysis. Am J Sports Med 1992;20:594–600.

[22] Horstman JK, Kantor GS, Samuelson KM. Investigation of lateral ankle ligament reconstruction. Foot Ankle 1981;1:338–42.

[23] Smith PA, Miller SJ, Berni AJ. A modified Chrisman-Snook procedure for reconstruction of the lateral ligaments of the ankle: review of 18 cases. Foot Ankle Int 1995;16:259–66.

[24] Acevedo JI, Myerson MS. Modification of the Chrisman-Snook technique. Foot Ankle Int 2000;21:154–5.

[25] Brostrom L. Sprained ankles. VI. Surgical treatment of "chronic" ligament ruptures. Acta Chir Scand 1966;132:551–65.

[26] Brostrom L. Sprained ankles. V. Treatment and prognosis in recent ligament ruptures. Acta Chir Scand 1966;132:537–50.

[27] Brostrom L. Sprained ankles. 3. Clinical observations in recent ligament ruptures. Acta Chir Scand 1965;130:560–9.

[28] Gould N. Repair of lateral ligament of ankle. Foot Ankle 1987;8:55–8.

[29] Bell SJ, Mologne TS, Sitler DF, et al. Twenty-six-year results after Brostrom procedure for chronic lateral ankle instability. Am J Sports Med 2006;34(6):975–8.

[30] Letts M, Davidson D, Mukhtar I. Surgical management of chronic lateral ankle instability in adolescents. J Pediatr Orthop 2003;23:392–7.

[31] Sugimoto K, Takakura Y, Kumai T, et al. Reconstruction of the lateral ankle ligaments with bone–patellar tendon graft in patients with chronic ankle instability: a preliminary report. Am J Sports Med 2002;30:340–6.

[32] Myerson M. Reconstructive foot and ankle surgery. Philadelphia (PA): Elsevier-Saunders; 2005.

[33] Sarrafian SK. Anatomy of the foot and ankle: descriptive, topographic, functional. Philadelphia (PA): JB Lippincott; 1983.

[34] Hintermann B. Biomechanics of the unstable ankle joint and clinical implications. Med Sci Sports Exerc 1999;31:S459–69.

[35] Lassiter TE Jr, Malone TR, Garrett WE Jr. Injury to the lateral ligaments of the ankle. Orthop Clin North Am 1989;20:629–40.

[36] Keener BJ, Sizensky JA. The anatomy of the calcaneus and surrounding structures. Foot Ankle Clin 2005;10:413–24.

[37] Leardini A, O'Connor JJ, Catani F, et al. A geometric model of the human ankle joint. J Biomech 1999;32:585–91.

[38] Milner CE, Soames RW. Anatomy of the collateral ligaments of the human ankle joint. Foot Ankle Int 1998;19:757–60.

[39] Burks RT, Morgan J. Anatomy of the lateral ankle ligaments. Am J Sports Med 1994;22: 72–7.

[40] Heilman AE, Braly WG, Bishop JO, et al. An anatomic study of subtalar instability. Foot Ankle 1990;10:224–8.

[41] Sosna A, Cech O. Anatomical bases for the reconstruction of fractures and ligament injuries in the region of the ankle joint. Acta Chir Orthop Traumatol Cech 1977;44: 288–303.

[42] Harper M. The lateral ligamentous support of the subtalar joint. Foot Ankle 1991;11:354–8.

[43] Aktan Ikiz ZA, Ucerler H, Bilge O. The anatomic features of the sural nerve with an emphasis on its clinical importance. Foot Ankle Int 2005;26:560–7.

[44] Stormont DM, Morrey BF, An KN, et al. Stability of the loaded ankle. Relation between articular restraint and primary and secondary static restraints. Am J Sports Med 1985;13: 295–300.

[45] Sommer C, Hintermann B, Nigg BM, et al. Influence of ankle ligaments on tibial rotation: an in vitro study. Foot Ankle Int 1996;17:79–84.

[46] Close JR, Inman VT, Poor PM, et al. The function of the subtalar joint. Clin Orthop Relat Res 1967;50:159–79.

[47] Inman VT. The human foot. Manit Med Rev 1966;46:513–5.

[48] Rasmussen O. Stability of the ankle joint. Analysis of the function and traumatology of the ankle ligaments. Acta Orthop Scand Suppl 1985;211:1–75.

[49] Attarian DE, McCrackin HJ, DeVito DP, et al. Biomechanical characteristics of human ankle ligaments. Foot Ankle 1985;6:54–8.

[50] Siegler S, Block J, Schneck CD. The mechanical characteristics of the collateral ligaments of the human ankle joint. Foot Ankle 1988;8:234–42.

[51] Attarian DE, McCrackin HJ, Devito DP, et al. A biomechanical study of human lateral ankle ligaments and autogenous reconstructive grafts. Am J Sports Med 1985;13:377–81.

[52] Kjaersgaard-Andersen P, Wethelund JO, Nielsen S. Lateral talocalcaneal instability following section of the calcaneofibular ligament: a kinesiologic study. Foot Ankle 1987;7:355–61.

[53] Cass JR, Settles H. Ankle instability: in vitro kinematics in response to axial load. Foot Ankle Int 1994;15:134–40.

[54] Boardman DL, Liu SH. Contribution of the anterolateral joint capsule to the mechanical stability of the ankle. Clin Orthop 1997;341:224–32.

[55] Hintermann B, Sommer C, Nigg B. The influence of ligament transection on tibial and calcaneal rotation with loading and dorsi-plantarflexion. Foot Ankle Int 1995;16:567–71.

[56] Bahr R, Pena F, Shine J, et al. Biomechanics of ankle ligament reconstruction. An in vitro comparison of the Brostrom repair, Watson-Jones reconstruction, and a new anatomic reconstruction technique. Am J Sports Med 1997;25:424–32.

[57] Colville MR. Surgical treatment of the unstable ankle. J Am Acad Orthop Surg 1998;6: 368–77.

[58] Liu SH, Baker CL. Comparison of lateral ankle ligamentous reconstruction procedures. Am J Sports Med 1994;22:313–7.

[59] Freeman MA, Dean MR, Hanham IW. The etiology and prevention of functional instability of the foot. J Bone Joint Surg Br 1965;47:678–85.

[60] Alanen J, Orava S, Heinonen OJ, et al. Peroneal tendon injuries. Report of thirty-eight operated cases. Ann Chir Gynaecol 2001;90:43–6.

[61] Fortin PT, Guettler J, Manoli A 2nd. Idiopathic cavovarus and lateral ankle instability: recognition and treatment implications relating to ankle arthritis. Foot Ankle Int 2002;23: 1031–7.

[62] Larsen E, Angermann P. Association of ankle instability and foot deformity. Acta Orthop Scand 1990;61:136–9.

[63] Tohyama H, Yasuda K, Ohkoshi Y, et al. Anterior drawer test for acute anterior talofibular ligament injuries of the ankle. How much load should be applied during the test? Am J Sports Med 2003;31:226–32.

[64] Seligson D, Gassman J, Pope M. Ankle instability: evaluation of the lateral ligaments. Am J Sports Med 1980;8:39–42.

[65] Laurin C, Mathieu J. Sagittal mobility of the normal ankle. Clin Orthop Relat Res 1975;99–104.

[66] Grace DL. Lateral ankle ligament injuries. Inversion and anterior stress radiography. Clin Orthop Relat Res 1984;153–9.

[67] Glasgow M, Jackson A, Jamieson AM. Instability of the ankle after injury to the lateral ligament. J Bone Joint Surg Br 1980;62-B:196–200.

[68] Louwerens JW, Ginai AZ, van Linge B, et al. Stress radiography of the talocrural and subtalar joints. Foot Ankle Int 1995;16:148–55.

[69] Frost SC, Amendola A. Is stress radiography necessary in the diagnosis of acute or chronic ankle instability? Clin J Sport Med 1999;9:40–5.

[70] Kerkhoffs GM, Blankevoort L, Sierevelt IN, et al. Two ankle joint laxity testers: reliability and validity. Knee Surg Sports Traumatol Arthrosc 2005;13:699–705.

[71] Hackenbruch W, Karpf PM. Injuries of the capsular ligament of the ankle joint, so-called "ankle joint distorsion." Fortschr Med 1977;95:1599–605.

[72] Karlsson J, Eriksson BI, Renstrom PA. Subtalar ankle instability. A review. Sports Med 1997;24:337–46.

[73] Gould N, Seligson D, Gassman J. Early and late repair of lateral ligament of the ankle. Foot Ankle 1980;1:84–9.

[74] Girard P, Anderson RB, Davis WH, et al. Clinical evaluation of the modified Brostrom-Evans procedure to restore ankle stability. Foot Ankle Int 1999;20:246–52.

[75] Coughlin MJ, Schenck RC Jr, Grebing BR, et al. Comprehensive reconstruction of the lateral ankle for chronic instability using a free gracilis graft. Foot Ankle Int 2004;25:231–41.

[76] Messer TM, Cummins CA, Ahn J, et al. Outcome of the modified Brostrom procedure for chronic lateral ankle instability using suture anchors. Foot Ankle Int 2000;21: 996–1003.

[77] Hennrikus WL, Mapes RC, Lyons PM, et al. Outcomes of the Chrisman-Snook and modified-Brostrom procedures for chronic lateral ankle instability. A prospective, randomized comparison. Am J Sports Med 1996;24:400–4.

[78] Karlsson J, Eriksson BI, Bergsten T, et al. Comparison of two anatomic reconstructions for chronic lateral instability of the ankle joint. Am J Sports Med 1997;25:48–53.

[79] Hamilton WG, Thompson FM, Snow SW. The modified Brostrom procedure for lateral ankle instability. Foot Ankle 1993;14:1–7.

ELSEVIER
SAUNDERS

Foot Ankle Clin N Am
11 (2006) 567–583

FOOT AND
ANKLE CLINICS

Operative Management of Chronic Ankle Instability: Plantaris Graft

Geert I. Pagenstert, MD*, Beat Hintermann, MD, Markus Knupp, MD

Department of Orthopaedic Surgery, Orthopaedic Clinic, University of Basel, Kantonsspital Liestal, CH-4410 Liestal, Switzerland

Many techniques are available for surgical reconstruction of chronic lateral ankle instability [1]. Nonanatomic procedures (or tenodesis procedures) cause numerous adverse effects [1,2], with restriction of motion of the subtalar and ankle joints and arthritis in up to 60% of patients [3]. The procedures that use the tip of the fibula or the posterior aspect of the fibula for insertion of the calcaneofibular ligament are nonanatomic, and act as tenodesis procedures. Precise reconstruction of anatomy is the key to successful lateral ligament reconstruction. The plantaris tendon offers the opportunity to use local autograft tissue with high tensile strength [4], a long graft when harvested at the proximal calf [5], and without the further damage to the impaired lateral muscular control intrinsic in peroneal tendon harvesting [6].

Ankle ligament injuries are the most common injuries in sports and recreational activities [6,7]. Acute lateral ankle sprains are optimally managed by functional rehabilitation [6,8–10], and surgery does not improve results [6,11]. Twenty percent to 40% of these patients will develop chronic instability and subsequent disability [6,12]. In most patients, late repair of the lateral ligaments is possible. If there are insufficient local tissue remnants, autografts, allografts, or synthetic substitutes can be used for ligament reconstruction, and 90% to 95% of these patients can be operated upon satisfactorily [13].

Controversies persist regarding anatomy and function of the lateral ankle ligaments despite concise anatomic and biomechanical studies. Consequently, nonanatomic ligament reconstructions techniques are still frequently used, and may explain postoperative problems, including persistent objective or subjective instability, pain, stiffness, development of arthritis,

---

* Corresponding author.
E-mail address: geert.pagenstert@ksli.ch (G.I. Pagenstert).

1083-7515/06/$ - see front matter © 2006 Elsevier Inc. All rights reserved.
doi:10.1016/j.fcl.2006.05.002 *foot.theclinics.com*

or decreased range of motion. This article describes the technique and clinical results of the senior author's ligament reconstruction procedure [14].

The choice of graft tissue for ligament reconstruction has less influence on the clinical outcome of lateral ankle ligament reconstruction than has anatomic versus nonanatomic reconstruction. Thus, graft selection often depends on the preference of the surgeon, and less on graft considerations. However, there are advantages and disadvantages of each graft and harvesting procedures. This article describes the advantages using the plantaris tendon autograft, and demonstrates the advantages using the author's harvesting procedure with a singe incision at the proximal calf [5].

Chronic lateral instability of the ankle

Clinical symptoms

Diagnosis is based on medical history and clinical findings. Patients complain of insecurity, instability, and giving way on uneven ground with difficulties in sports or daily activities, with recurrent sprains, pain, tenderness, and at times bruising over the lateral aspect of the ankle [15–17]. Approximately 30% of patients may be asymptomatic between the events, and others may present with chronic lateral pain, tenderness, swelling, or giving way [15]. We test ankle laxity with the patient sitting with the legs hanging free. This will prevent reactive muscular stabilization by involuntary peroneal muscle contraction [18]. Talar tilt test or anterior drawer sign are positive in patients with structural ligament insufficiency, whereas these tests may be negative when only functional ankle instability is present [19]. Functional ankle instability is likely caused by damaged mechanoreceptors in the lateral ligaments. It is diagnosed with gait analysis or prolonged peroneal muscle reaction time with electromyographic measurements [20–22]. After intensive physical therapy, surgery may be suggested in chronic functional instability in patients with, and probably also without, combined mechanical instability [1].

Imaging

The finding of laxity may be documented by forced inversion or anterior drawer films. A talar tilt of more than 5° difference to the contralateral uninjured ankle is usually considered pathologic [23], although others claim a minimum of 10° [24,25]. Anterior subluxation of over 6 mm is usually considered pathologic [23]. However, wide variations of up to 25° of talar tilt and differences from side to side of up to 19° have been found to be present in about 5% of the population [24]. Hence, radiographic assessment of lateral laxity is highly unreliable. This becomes even more evident, as only 40% of the patients demonstrating radiographic instability will have symptoms of an unstable ankle [26]. Approximately the same percentage of patients with symptomatic ankle instability will demonstrate no laxity on stress radiographs [25].

Anatomy of the two major lateral ankle ligaments

Anterior talofibular ligament

The anterior talofibular ligament (ATFL) blends with the anterior capsule of the ankle, and spans the anterolateral aspect of the ankle joint. The ligament originates at the anterior edge of the fibula, just lateral to the articular cartilage of the lateral malleolus. The center of attachment lies 10 mm proximal to the tip of the fibula when measured along the long axis of the fibula. The insertion on the talus begins directly distal to the articular surface, and the center is 18 mm proximal to the subtalar joint [18,27]. The ATFL is the first ligament restricting supination of the foot, and is most frequently injured in ankle sprains. Chronic insufficiency of the ATFL is typically combined with a pathologic anterior drawer sign. When the deltoid ligament is intact, pathologic internal rotation of the talus is noted when performing the anterior drawer test. [9] Nearly all surgical procedures for lateral ankle instability include the reconstruction of the ATFL.

Calcaneofibular ligament

Contrary to popular belief, the calcaneofibular ligament (CFL) does not originate from the apex of the tip of the lateral malleolus. Its attachment on the anterior edge of distal fibula is centered 8.5 mm from the distal tip just below the origin of the ATFL. The ligament courses medially, posteriorly, and inferiorly from its fibular origin to the cacaneal insertion. The calcaneal insertion begins 13 mm distal to the subtalar joint with its proximal edge on a line nearly perpendicular to the subtalar joint [14,27].

The CFL effectively spans the ankle and subtalar joints, which have markedly different axes of rotation [23,28–31]. Thus, this ligament must be attached so that it does not restrict motion of either joint, whether they move independently or simultaneously. When projected onto the sagittal plane of the subtalar joint axis, the ligament parallels this axis. When projected onto a vertical transverse plane, the ligament diverges from the subtalar axis at an acute angle [32].

The angle between the CFL and ATFL was measured on 50 cadavers. In the sagittal plane, the average angle was 105° (range 70–140°). In the coronal plane, the average angle was 100° (range 60–140°) [32]. The CFL resists ankle and subtalar joint supination, restricting inversion and internal rotation of the subtalar joint. Strain in the CFL increases with dosiflexion when it becomes more vertically orientated, and takes over the role as the lateral collateral ligament of the ankle. Chronic insufficiency of the CFL is typically combined with a pathologic talar tilt test in neutral ankle position. During ankle dorsiflexion, the fibula moves posteriorly, the talus glides anteriorly using the medial malleolus as a central pivot, and the syndesmotic ligaments are taut [18,33,34]. Reconstructive procedures using tenodesis procedures or the tip or the posterior edge of the fibula prevent subtalar rotation and posterior fibula motion with ankle dorsiflexion. This tight lateral ankle construct changes the physiologic center of rotation of the ankle from medial to lateral, disturbing the coupling mechanism between leg and foot, causing subtalar and ankle arthritis [3,29].

Biomechanics of the lateral ankle ligaments

Stabilizing function of ankle ligaments

Each of the lateral ligaments has a role in stabilizing the ankle or subtalar joint, depending on the position of the foot. In dorsiflexion, the posterior talofibular ligament is maximally stressed and the CFL is taut, whereas the ATFL is loose. Conversely, in plantarflexion, the ATFL is taut and the CFL and posterior talofibular ligaments become loose [35,36]. Some variation to this is allowed by the different patterns of divergence between the anterior talofibular and CFLs.

The CFL retains its parallelism to the axis of the subtalar joint as the ankle passes from plantarflexion to dorsiflexion. In plantarflexion, both the ligament and the subtalar joint axis become horizontal. In dorsiflexion, both the ligament and the subtalar joint axis approach a more vertical position. Thus, in dorsiflexion, the CFL can act as a true collateral ligament and prevent talar tilt. As the ankle joint goes from dorsiflexion to plantarfelxion, the CFL is less able to resist talar tilt, and the ATFL functions as collateral ligament to resist talar tilt, and vice versa [32].

Sequential sectioning of the lateral ligaments has demonstrated the function of these ligaments at different ankle positions and at various loading conditions. Johnson and Markolf [37] studied the laxity of the ankle after sectioning the ATFL: most changes occurred in plantarflexion, with smaller changes in laxity in dorsiflexion. This suggests that the ATFL limits talar tilt throughout motion but has greatest advantage in plantarflexion. Rasmussen and Tovberg-Jensen [38] further confirmed the above findings: talar tilt is limited in plantarflexion and in neutral position by the ATFL, and in dorsiflexion by the CFL plus the posterior talofibular ligament. Hollis and colleagues [39], in a similar in vitro study, found that inversion motion of the ankle increases when sectioning the CFL in addition to the ATFL.

The cadaveric sudies of Kjaersgaard-Andersen and colleagues [40,41] showed a 20% increase in rotation of the subtalar (talocalcaneal) joint, and a 61% to 77% increase in talocalcaneal adduction after release of the CFL. Heilman and colleagues [42] performed a similar cadaver study with sequential release of the CFL, the lateral capsule, and the interosseous talocalcaneal ligament. They documented a 5-mm opening between the posterior facets of the talus and calcaneous with a stress radiograph after release of the CFL, and an increase of 7 mm when the talocalcaneal ligament was also sectioned.

The role that the lateral talocalcaneal ligament plays in subtalar instability is not completely understood. It is possible that CFL injury may result in greater instability for an individual lacking a talocalcaneal ligament compared with an inividual who has an intact lateral talocalcaneal ligament. Loss of the CFL would comprise subtalar stability more if there were no separate lateral talocalcaneal ligament [27].

Kinematics of ankle instability

Motion between the tibia and the foot is a complex combination of ankle and subtalar motion limited by osseous shape and soft tissue interaction. Ankle motion does not occur around one single axis [27,29,43–45]. Rather, ankle motion combines dorsiflexion and plantarflexion with internal and external rotation and some anterior/posterior translation of the talus on the tibia [28,44,45]. Many studies have tried to elucidate how the ligaments contribute to this functional interplay with the bone structures [30,46–51]. Most reports focus on the lateral ligaments and the role they play in maintaining lateral ankle stability [31,36,38,52]. Some have tried to determine the amount of tilting that occurs after selective release of the anterior talofibular, calcaneofibular, posterior talofibular, and deltoid ligament [31,46,51,52]. Although the magnitude of tilt has been shown to vary significantly [46], some tilt does occur with the loss of these ligaments [19,31,36]. These measurements of talar tilt, however, do not provide information about the rotational instability that is created by the ligament release. Thus, despite the vast amount of literature, the debate continues over the instability being one of tilting the talus in the mortise of one of axial rotation, or both.

Coupling mechanism between foot and leg

We studied the role of the ankle ligaments in the coupling mechanism between foot and leg, especially in transferring movement between calcaneal and tibial rotation [44]. Section of the lateral ligaments did not significantly affect the tibial rotation and foot eversion–inversion for a given dorsiplantarflexion. If the deltoid ligament was also sectioned, however, the physiologic pattern of motion was greatly altered, especially on plantarflexion. From this, the transfer mechanism at the ankle joint complex does markedly depend on the integrity of the deltoid ligament [45]. One explanation may be the inconstant axis of rotation of the talus in the mortise, as the talus rotates around a variable axis in all three planes, given that the trochlea has a conical instead of a cylindrical shape, using the medial malleolus as center of rotation (central joint pivot) [32–34,43].

Rotational instability

Studying the passive rotational stability of the loaded ankle, Fraser and Ahmed [47] found that with increasing load, rotation decreased. McCullough and Burge [48] investigated the internal/external rotation of the ankle with application of an axial load. They also noted that increasing the axial load decreased the axial rotation when the ankle ligaments were intact as well as when the ankle ligaments were sectioned. Stormont and colleagues [51] evaluated the effects of lateral ligament sectioning in a preloaded model and found that the articular surfaces supplied 30% of the stability in rotation and 100% of the stability in inversion testing. However, in the two latter studies, rotation occurred only about one axis: ether leg rotation was allowed and eversion/inversion constrained, or vice versa. The data from these two studies should, therefore, be cautiously applied to the in vivo situation of ankle instability. Indeed, both ankle and subtalar motion required rotation about all three reference axes [32], and, if external rotation is restricted, talar tilt will likewise be limited [52].

Cass and Settles [46] studied the kinematics of ankle instability after lateral ligament sectioning in a model where axial rotation was not constrained. They found no tilting of the talus in the mortise to occur with isolated release of the ATFL or CFL. After both ligaments were released, an average talar tilt of 20.6° occurred. External rotation of the leg occurred with inversion averaging 11.1° in the intact specimen. The leg averaged a further external rotation of 4.9° after ATFL release and 12.8° further than the intact inverted specimen when the CFL in addition had been released. Therefore, the ATLF and the CFL work together to prevent tilting of the talus, and that the articular surfaces do not seem to prevent tilting of the talus in the mortise. Obviously, talar tilt does occur with inversion even in the presence of an axial load [46,53]. Inversion is accompanied by a obligatory external rotation of the leg [32,52–54]. In intact specimens, external rotation occurs at the subtalar joint [46,53]. After loss of ligamentous support, external rotation increases, but not at the subtalar joint [45,46]. Rather, this increase occurs between the tibia and the talus. One may thus speculate that ankle laxity, at least in one form, is an axial rotational one.

This rotational concept may explain why symptoms of ankle instability occur in the absence of radiographically demonstrable talar tilt. Another factor that may be taken into account is the role of the subtalar joint in ankle instability [41,55].

Recent in vitro studies support the hypothesis that, in addition to maintaining lateral ankle stability, the lateral ankle ligaments play a significant role in rotational ankle stability. The loss of the ATFL an/or the CFL leads to a measurable increase in inversion without any tilting of the talus or subtalar gapping. Also, loss of ATFL function does increase external rotation of the leg. The loss of ATFL restraint, in fact, unlocks the subtalar joint, allowing further inversion. This increase in inversion may lead to symptomatic instability. If this were true, no tilting would be necessary at either ankle or subtalar levels to induce structural instability.

These rotational concepts may explain why repair of the ATFL alone can provide successful clinical results for treatment of ankle instability [15,56]. It may also explain why reconstructions that simply tenodese the fifth metatarsal to the fibula, thereby preventing external rotation, are sufficient to mange ankle instability [57]. Most common tenodesis procedures [56–60], however, significantly restrict subtalar motion, and thus alter the mechanical interplay of ankle and subtalar motion. When surgical repair of the CFL is directed to stabilize the subtalar joint, this ligament must be attached in such a way that motion is not restricted in either joint, whether they move independently or simultaneously.

Conclusion and clinical implications

Precise anatomic and biomechanical understanding led to a modified routing procedure for lateral ankle reconstruction. Great attention is paid not to disturb the movement transfer between the leg and foot by stabilizing talar tilt and excessive talar internal rotation. A key feature is the isometric fixation of the conjoined insertion of ATFL and CFL to the anterior aspect of the fibula. Thus, the CFL stays parallel to the axis of the subtalar joint during the full excursion of range of motion. This allows simultaneous and isolated movement of the subtalar and ankle joints without changing the central pivot at the medial malleolus.

Anatomic reconstruction of lateral ankle ligaments using plantaris autograft

General or spinal anesthesia or a Bier's block is offered according to the patients wishes, although we do not recommend a Bier's block because harvesting the plantaris tendon is more difficult. The patient is placed supine with a pillow or sandbag under the ipsilateral hip to tilt 30° the affected site. The leg is exsanguinated, and a tourniquet is inflated. When general or spinal anesthesia is used, the tourniquet is placed 15 cm proximal to the knee. If a Bier's block is used, the tourniquet is placed below the knee. Arthroscopy with manual distraction is performed via a single anterior portal between the tibialis anterior and extensor hallucis longus tendons. The ankle and subtalar ligaments and cartilages are evaluated, and additional surgery is planned according to these findings.

An incision is made from the tip of the lateral malleolus 4 to 6 cm toward the base of the fifth metatarsal with the foot held in plantarflexion. The ventral part of the malleolus is exposed with the conjoined ligament insertion of the CFL and ATFL and the joint capsule. In the distal part of the incision, the sinus tarsi of the subtalar joint is opened, and any scar tissue is debrided, as it can be a source of pain. The ankle is opened along the ventral boarder parallel to the possible remnants of the talofibular ligament. The peroneal tendons within their sheath are dissected at the distal to posterior aspect of the malleolus, and the tendons retracted with a right angle retractor to evaluate the CFL to its insertions. After thorough evaluation of these two major stabilizing ligaments, a decision on how to proceed is made. If the local tissue available is less than 50%, or not adequate to the demands of the patient, we use a free tendon graft. In active patients or in failed previous repair, tendon augmentation is routinely undertaken. A wet swab is placed in the ankle incision, and the tendon of plantaris harvested.

The plantaris tendon can be harvested at the ankle joint level just medial to the Achilles tendon at the tuber calcanei with at least one 2-cm to 7-cm skin incision [14,56,61,62]. Failure to locate the tendon is reported in 12% to 20% of patients [14,56,61,62], although cadaver and MRI or ultrasound studies show absence of the plantaris tendon in only 6% to 7% of patients [63–65]. This reflects the difficulties with this approach. Commonly, adhesions with the Achilles tendon at its insertion on the calcaneus or with the intermuscular fascia make identification of the plantaris tendon difficult [63,65]. In addition, the insertion may be located at the bursa calcanei, flexor retinaculum, ankle joint capsule, or simply confluent with the intermuscular fascia in the distal few centimeters [65,66]. Moreover cases of painful scar formation occurred because the distal incision is located in the area where footwear pressure is exerted.

As the plantaris longus tendon runs at the medial border of the triceps surae in the proximal calf (Fig. 1) [66], our preferred technique uses an incision at the medial boarder of the triceps surae 25 cm to 30 cm proximal to the medial malleolus. A 2-cm longitudinal incision is made (Fig. 2a). Subcutaneous blunt dissection to the fascia is performed protecting the saphenous nerve and vein. Again, a 2-cm longitudinal incision is made in the fascia to allow the surgeon's finger to enter the intermuscular space between the soleus and gastrocnemius muscle (Fig. 2b). The only rigid tubular structure that is palpable at this muscular interspace is the plantaris tendon. The tendon is further developed with the finger or a nerve retractor (Fig. 2c). After fixing the tendon with a clamp it is cut and anchored with a Bunnell stitch technique with a 0 atraumatic absorbable stitch. With a blunt tendon stripper the plantaris tendon is dissected in distal direction. The tendon stripper is introduced and advanced keeping the tendon under tension. At the level of the ankle joint, the inner cylinder of the stripper is rotated, cutting the tendon without additional skin incisions. The tendon is stored in a wet sponge for later use. Wound closure is performed with a subcuticular running stitch. Wound tension is neutralized with sterile strips to achieve a favorable cosmetic result.

Bony tunnels 3.2 mm in diameter are placed around the anatomic insertions of the ATFL and CFL. With absent remnants, precise knowledge of the anatomy of the ankle is the key to reconstructive techniques. Two tunnels 10-mm deep are drilled in an anteroposterior direction into the anterior

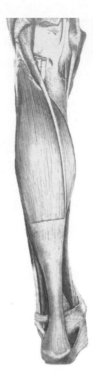

Fig. 1. Between the gastrocnemius and soleus there is only one tubular structure: the plantaris tendon. No vessels or nerves can be injured during blunt dissection to identify the plantaris tendon.

aspect of the fibula 7 and 13 mm proximal to the distal tip of the lateral malleolus, respectively (Fig. 3). In addition, these tunnels are placed just at the bony border to the fibular cartilage. The two tunnels are directed posteriorly to join each other within the fibula at a depth of 10 mm. From the posterolateral aspect of the fibula, an additional tunnel is drilled to meet the anterior tunnels at the site where they join (Fig. 3). A Weber's reduction clamp is inserted and swiveled through the holes to smoothen the sharp edges of the osseous channels and make sure of their continuity (Fig. 3). Two tunnels are drilled in the talus in the same fashion 14 and 22 mm cranial to the subtalar joint, at the former site of ligament insertion, just distal to the cartilaginous surface of the talus with a craniocaudal distance of 6 mm to 8 mm to each other, again in a converging fashion. Convergence should occur approximately 18 mm cranial to the subtalar joint. Again, the Weber's clamp is used to smoothen and assure continuity of the channels. Another tunnel is produced parallel to the posterior facet of the calcaneus at the insertion site of CFL, approximately 13 mm distal to it, on a line perpendicular to the subtalar joint. During the later procedure, the peroneal tendons are gently retracted.

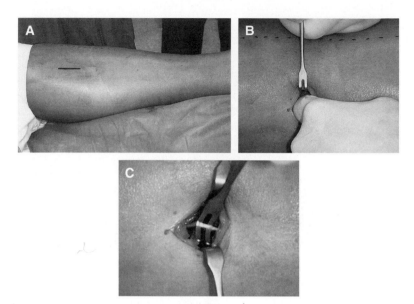

Fig. 2. (*A*) Overview and skin incision to harvest the plantaris longus tendon. (*B*) Blunt dissection between the soleus and gastrocnemius muscles. (*C*) Tendon developed with a nerve retractor. The average length of the harvested tendon is 30 cm.

The plantaris tendon graft is directed through the holes with the foot held in supination and dorsiflexion (Fig. 4a–g), and sutured to itself and the periosteum with the anchor stitch holding the tendon under slight tension. Alternatively, or in addition, small interference screws can be used in the

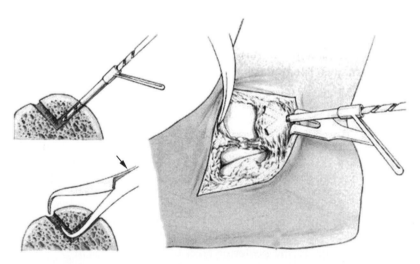

Fig. 3. The surgeon uses a ruler to locate the ligamentous insertions and to place the drill holes in a converging direction. Swiveling action of the Weber's clamp assures continuity of the channels and smoothens the osseous sharp edges.

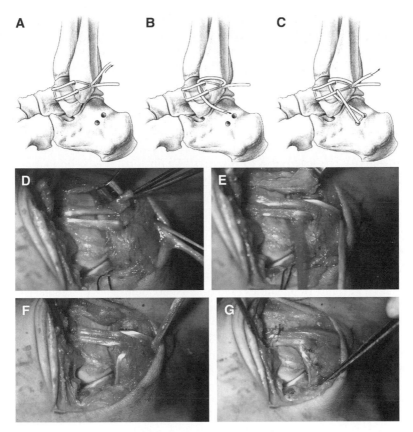

Fig. 4. (*A, D*) Routing of the plantaris tendon first through the fibula to the talus and back. (*B, E*) The second portion of the plantaris tendon is folded over the reconstructed ATLF and guided medially to the calcaneus. This shifts the reconstructed CFL more medial in respect to its insertion at the fibula. This enables the CFL to stay parallel to the subtalar joint during range of motion. (*C, F*) The CFL is reconstructed, and the tension is equally distributed after taking the foot through a full range of motion. (*G*) Appearance before wound closure.

talus and calcaneus. No additional interference screws is used in the fibula to allow gliding adaptation of graft tension during range of motion. The construct is then checked for evenly distributed tension and unimpeded ankle and subtalar joint mobility. Additional No. 0 absorbable suture may be necessary to enhance the construction with the remnants of the fibula ligaments or extensor retinaculum. The peroneal tendons are relocated in the posterior aspect of the fibula, and the peroneal sheath is closed. After skin closure and compressive dressing, the ankle is placed in a neutral splint.

Postoperative management

Postoperatively, the lower leg is immobilized in a removable soft cast with the ankle in neutral for 2 to 4 weeks at night. Cautious range of motion for dorsi- and plantar flexion is allowed after 2 to 3 days, with isometric training of all lower leg muscles. Eversion and inversion, supination, and pronation are permitted 4 to 6 weeks postoperatively. Orthopedic boots (Ortho-Rehab, Künzli AG, CH-5210 Windisch, Switzerland) or semirigid ankle braces preventing eversion, inversion, and excessive dorsi- and plantar flexion can be used, gradual weight bearing as tolerated is allowed after 2 to 3 days, and always reached after 10 days [67]. Return to work ability is allowed for sedentary workers after 10 days, and for heavy laborers after 4 to 6 weeks. Heavy laborers may use rigid protective footwear continuously. Sport activity is started at 4 to 6 weeks. Again, orthopedic boots or ankle braces should be worn, and gradually discarded to ensure that the reconstruction is not stressed abruptly. Return to full sports activity depends on each individual, but generally occurs at 4 to 12 weeks from the operation.

Results

Over 10 years, in 56 ankles the remnants of the ligaments were insufficient for primary repair. In 52 ankles (48 patients: 30 males and 18 females), a free plantaris tendon graft was used for anatomic ligament reconstruction as described above. The average age at operation was 28.6 years (range 16–46 years). The right ankle was affected 28 times, the left 24. The time between initial injury and operation was ranged between 9 months and 14 years (average 3.2 years). Three patients had had a ligament repair before. All remaining patients had undergone prolonged conservative management before the operation.

Forty-five patients with 49 ankles were controlled with an average follow up of 8.5 years (range 6–15 years). Three patients could not be located. Forty-four patients (98%) had no limitations of sports or everyday activity. Twelve patients reported inconstant discomfort, or mild swelling at the ankle was present after running or walking for more than 1 hour. Eleven of these patients showed no evidence of structural laxity at clinical testing and stress xradiographs. One patient reported mild insecurity playing soccer, with inconstant pain at the lateral ankle after an additional ankle sprain since the time of surgery. This patient had a positive anterior drawer sign and stress radiographs. The American Orthopaedic Foot and Ankle Society (AOFAS)-Hindfoot-Score revealed an average of 95.6 points (range 85–100). The AOFAS score was graded in 40 patients (82%) as excellent, in 8 patients (16%) good, in 1 patient as moderate, and in 0 patients unsatisfactory. Age, gender, sports activity, delay between injury and operation, or idiopathic joint laxity had had no influence on the outcome.

Range of motion for dorsi- and plantarflexion was unrestricted compared with the uninjured site. In two patients, supination (inversion) of the subtalar joint was mildly restricted compared with the uninjured site.

At the latest follow-up, 41 patients (44 ankles) undertook their previous sports at their preoperative level. Three patients (four ankles) had changed their previous sport or level for other reasons. One patient (one ankle) was not practicing sport as he did before surgery.

Once a patient has reached an excellent or good result, this was durable over time in all but one patient, with no worsening. In one patient, a new injury caused again lateral ankle instability. In no patient did sport participation level deteriorate. In no patient did work ability deteriorate.

Complications

Plantaris tendon harvesting produces negligible donor site morbidity [66]. In our series, the plantaris tendon was absent in three patients (5.3%) and too weak to serve as a graft in one patient (1.7%). If the tendon is absent, the long extensor tendons of the third or fourth toes can be used, with low donor site morbidity [68]. In 56 grafting procedures, we did not experience complications from harvesting of the plantaris tendon. Hematoma or neural injuries may occur due to the anatomic proximity of the saphenous vein and nerve over the medial aspect of the proximal calf.

Two patients had marked varus of the hindfoot, and a Dwyer osteotomy to reconstitute the normal hindfoot alignment was added. One of these two patients suffered a superficial wound infection which healed within 3 weeks with dressing and oral antibiotics. Three patients developed mild discomfort at their scars: two at the lateral ankle and one at the the the calf. No patient had to take pain medications.

If the tunnels for the osseous channels are not meeting each other or too much force is applied to the Weber's clamp, a cortical fracture of the fibula might be produced. We did not observe any of these complications.

Discussion

There are more than 60 different surgical procedures for the management of chronic lateral ankle instability [1], broadly classified into anatomic and nonanatomic [19]. The nonanatomic procedures are basically tenodesis procedures using exogenous or endogenous material. Exogenous material bears the risk of hypersensitivity, local inflammation, or infection. Endogenous materials are most often the peroneal tendons, frequently used for Watson-Jones, Chrisman-Snook, or Evans operation [1,2]. Even though good short-term results have been reported, the results deteriorate over time. Only 33% of patients who underwent Evans procedure resumed athletic activity, and only 50% had satisfactory results 14 years after surgery [2,3,69].

Numerous problems accompany tenodesis procedures: healing is prolonged, anatomy is not restored, peroneal tendons are damaged, and compromise to the active muscular stabilization system of the lateral ankle. All tenodesis procedures limit subtalar joint mobility; return to full activity is prolonged, and late occurrence of degenerative joint disease of the subtalar and ankle joints is found in over 60% of patients [2,3,70]. We believe that reconstructive procedures that use the tip or the posterior aspect of the fibula as insertion for the CFL should be considered as nonanatomic, as they produce a tenodesis-like limitation of ankle and subtalar joint function, with the sequelae described above.

Bohnsack and colleagues [4] tested frequently used autologous tissues used for lateral ligament reconstruction. The plantaris tendon showed the highest tensile strength (N/mm^3) compared with fascia lata, periostal flap, Achilles tendon, peroneus brevis, or longus tendons. With the authors' harvesting procedure, morbidity of the donor site and unavailability of the graft was markedly reduced. Using fascia lata or hamstring tendons require unnecessary enlargement of the surgical field to the knee or upper leg. Peroneals are best preserved for active dynamic stabilization of the ankle. Grafting further damages the impaired functional lateral ankle control. Periostal flaps contain predominantly unstructured soft tissue and vessels to nourish the bone. The potent periostal cells are thought to convert to structured collagen fibers within months. Primary stability is significant below all tendon autografts [4].

Summary

Precise knowledge of lateral ankle ligaments anatomy and biomechanics is mandatory for successful surgical reconstruction. The displayed reconstruction procedure fulfilled these requirements, and showed excellent clinical outcome.

The described harvesting of the plantaris tendon at the proximal calf allows the use of a relatively long tendon autograft compared with the traditional harvesting procedure at the os calcis. Consequently, this procedure gives the surgeon a more efficient access to a local tendon autograft for numerous surgical procedures in the field of foot and ankle surgery.

References

[1] Nyska M, Mann G, Hetsroni I, et al. Operative treatment of ankle instability: non-anatomic reconstructions. In: Chan KM, Karlsson J, editors. ISAKOS and FIMS world consensus conference on ankle instability. Stockholm, Sweden; 2005. p. 56–8.
[2] Karlsson J, Bergsten T, Lansinger O, et al. Lateral instability of the ankle treated by the Evans procedure. A long-term clinical and radiological follow-up. J Bone Joint Surg Br 1988;70(3):476–80.
[3] Krips R, Brandsson S, Swensson C, et al. Anatomical reconstruction and Evans tenodesis of the lateral ligaments of the ankle. Clinical and radiological findings after follow-up for 15 to 30 years. J Bone Joint Surg Br 2002;84(2):232–6.
[4] Bohnsack M, Surie B, Kirsch IL, et al. Biomechanical properties of commonly used autogenous transplants in the surgical treatment of chronic lateral ankle instability. Foot Ankle Int 2002;23(7):661–4.
[5] Pagenstert GI, Valderrabano V, Hintermann B. Lateral ankle ligament reconstruction with free plantaris tendon graft. Tech Foot Ankle Surg 2005;4(2):104–12.

[6] Chan KM, Karlsson J. ISAKOS and FIMS world consensus conference on ankle instability. Stockholm: Sweden; 2005.

[7] Garrick JG. The frequency of injurymechanism of injury and epidemiology of ankle sprains. Am J Sports Med 1977;5:241–2.

[8] Pijnenburg ACM, Dijk van CN, Bossuyt PMM, et al. Treatment for lateral ankle ligament ruptures: a meta-analysis. J Bone Joint Surg Am 2000;82:761–73.

[9] Nilsson S. Sprains of the lateral ankle ligaments. An epidemiologic and clinical study with special reference to different forms of conservative treatment. J Oslo City Hosp 1982;32:3–29.

[10] Eiff MP, Smith AT, Smith GE. Early mobilization versus immobilization in the treatment of lateral ankle sprains. Am J Sports Med 1994;22(1):83–8.

[11] Kerkhoffs GM, Handoll HH, de Bie R, et al. Surgical versus conservative treatment for acute injuries of the lateral ligament complex of the ankle in adults. Cochrane Database Syst Rev 2002;3:CD000380.

[12] Karlsson J, Lansinger O. Lateral instability of the ankle joint (1). Non-surgical treatment is the first choice—20 per cent may need ligament surgery. Lakartidningen 1991;88(15): 1399–402.

[13] Karlsson J. Ligament injuries of the ankle—what happens later? Non-surgical treatment is effective in 80–90 per cent of cases. Lakartidningen 1998;95(40):4376–8.

[14] Hintermann B, Renggli P. Anatomic reconstruction of the lateral ligaments of the ankle using a plantaris tendon graft in the treatment of chronic ankle joint instability. Orthopade 1999;28(9):778–84.

[15] Brostrom L. Sprained ankles—VI. Surgical treatment of "chronic" ligament ruptures. Acta Chir Scand 1966;132:551–65.

[16] Staples OS. Result study of ruptures of lateral ligaments of the ankle. Clin Orthop 1972;85: 50–8.

[17] Karlsson J, Bergsten T, Lansinger O, et al. Reconstruction of the lateral ligaments of the ankle for chronic lateral instability. J Bone Joint Surg Am 1988;70(4):581–8.

[18] Hintermann B. Biomechanics of the unstable ankle joint and clinical implications. Med Sci Sports Exerc 1999;31(7 Suppl):S459–69.

[19] Peters JW, Trevino SG, Renstrom PA. Chronic lateral ankle instability. Foot Ankle 1991; 12(3):182–91.

[20] Konradsen L, Ravn JB, Sorensen AI. Proprioception at the ankle: the effect of anaesthetic blockade of ligament receptors. J Bone Joint Surg Br 1993;75(3):433–6.

[21] Konradsen L. Sensori-motor control of the uninjured and injured human ankle. J Electromyogr Kinesiol 2002;12(3):199–203.

[22] Konradsen L, Ravn JB. Ankle instability caused by prolonged peroneal reaction time. Acta Orthop Scand 1990;61(5):388–90.

[23] Hintermann B, Holzach P, Matter P. Injury pattern of the fibular ligaments. Radiological diagnosis and clinical study. Unfallchirurg 1992;95(3):142–7.

[24] Drez D Jr, Young JC, Waldman D, et al. Nonoperative treatment of double lateral ligament tears of the ankle. Am J Sports Med 1982;10(4):197–200.

[25] Kristiansen B. Evans' repair of lateral instability of the ankle joint. Acta Orthop Scand 1981; 52(6):679–82.

[26] Freeman MA. Instability of the foot after injuries to the lateral ligament of the ankle. J Bone Joint Surg Br 1965;47(4):669–77.

[27] Burks RT, Morgan J. Anatomy of the lateral ankle ligaments. Am J Sports Med 1994;22: 72–7.

[28] Close JR. Some applications of the functional anatomy of the ankle joint. J Bone Joint Surg Am 1956;38-A(4):761–81.

[29] Hintermann B, Nigg BM. Movement transfer between foot and calf in vitro. Sportverletz Sportschaden 1994;8(2):60–6.

[30] Michelson JD, Clarke HJ, Jinnah RH. The effect of loading on tibiotalar alignment in cadaver ankles. Foot Ankle 1990;10(5):280–4.

[31] Larsen E. Experimental instability of the ankle. A radiographic investigation. Clin Orthop Relat Res 1986;204:193–200.

[32] Stiehl JB. Inman's joints of the ankle. 2nd ed. Baltimore (MD): Williams & Wilkins; 1991.

[33] Barnett CH, Napier JR. The axis of rotation at the ankle joint in man; its influence upon the form of the talus and the mobility of the fibula. J Anat 1952;86(1):1–9.

[34] Sammarco J. Biomechanics of the ankle. I. Surface velocity and instant center of rotation in the sagittal plane. Am J Sports Med 1977;5(6):231–4.

[35] Colville MR, Marder RA, Boyle JJ, et al. Strain measurement in lateral ankle ligaments. Am J Sports Med 1990;18(2):196–200.

[36] Renstrom PA, Wertz M, Incavo S, et al. Strain in the lateral ligaments of the ankle. Foot Ankle 1988;9:59–63.

[37] Johnson EE, Markolf KL. The contribution of the anterior talofibular ligament to ankle laxity. J Bone Joint Surg Am 1983;65(1):81–8.

[38] Rasmussen O, Tovborg-Jensen I. Mobility of the ankle joint: recording of rotatory movements in the talocrural joint in vitro with and without the lateral collateral ligaments of the ankle. Acta Orthop Scand 1982;53(1):155–60.

[39] Hollis JM, Blasier RD, Flahiff CM. Simulated lateral ankle ligamentous injury. Change in ankle stability. Am J Sports Med 1995;23(6):672–7.

[40] Kjaersgaard-Andersen P, Wethelund JO, Nielsen S. Lateral talocalcaneal instability following section of the calcaneofibular ligament: a kinesiologic study. Foot Ankle 1987;7(6): 355–61.

[41] Kjaersgaard-Andersen P, Wethelund JO, Helmig P, et al. Effect of the calcaneofibular ligament on hindfoot rotation in amputation specimens. Acta Orthop Scand 1987;58(2): 135–8.

[42] Heilman AE, Braly WG, Bishop JO, et al. An anatomic study of subtalar instability. Foot Ankle 1990;10(4):224–8.

[43] Hicks JH. The mechanics of the foot. I. The joints. J Anat 1953;87:345–57.

[44] Sommer C, Hintermann B, Nigg BM, et al. Influence of ankle ligaments on tibial rotation: an in vitro study. Foot Ankle Int 1996;17(2):79–84.

[45] Hintermann B, Sommer C, Nigg BM. Influence of ligament transection on tibial and calcaneal rotation with loading and dorsi-plantarflexion. Foot Ankle Int 1995;16(9):567–71.

[46] Cass JR, Settles H. Ankle instability: in vitro kinematics in response to axial load. Foot Ankle Int 1994;15(3):134–40.

[47] Fraser GA, Ahmed AM. Passive rotational stability of the weight bearing talocrural joint: an in vitro biomechanical study. Orthop Trans 1983;7:248.

[48] McCullough CJ, Burge PD. Rotatory stability of the load-bearing ankle. An experimental study. J Bone Joint Surg Br 1980;62-B(4):460–4.

[49] Nigg BM, Skarvan G, Frank CB, et al. Elongation and forces of ankle ligaments in a physiological range of motion. Foot Ankle 1990;11(1):30–40.

[50] Parlasca R, Shoji H, D'Ambrosia RD. Effects of ligamentous injury on ankle and subtalar joints: a kinematic study. Clin Orthop Relat Res 1979;140:266–72.

[51] Stormont DM, Morrey BF, An KN, et al. Stability of the loaded ankle. Relation between articular restraint and primary and secondary static restraints. Am J Sports Med 1985; 13(5):295–300.

[52] Laurin CA, Ouellet R, St Jacques R. Talar and subtalar tilt: an experimental investigation. Can J Surg 1968;11(3):270–9.

[53] Lundberg A, Svensson OK, Nemeth G, et al. The axis of rotation of the ankle joint. J Bone Joint Surg Br 1989;71(1):94–9.

[54] Hintermann B, Nigg BM. In vitro kinematics of the axially loaded ankle complex in response to dorsiflexion and plantarflexion. Foot Ankle Int 1995;16(8):514–8.

[55] Clanton TO. Instability of the subtalar joint. Orthop Clin North Am 1989;20(4):583–92.

[56] Weber BG, Hupfauer W. Zur Behandlung der frischen fibularen Bandruptur und der chronischen fibularen Bandinsuffizienz. Arch Orthop Trauma Surg 1969;65:251–7.

[57] Cass JR, Morrey BF, Chao EY. Three-dimensional kinematics of ankle instability following serial sectioning of lateral collateral ligaments. Foot Ankle 1984;5(3):142–9.

[58] Snook GA, Chrisman OD, Wilson TC. Long-term results of the Chrisman-Snook operation for reconstruction of the lateral ligaments of the ankle. J Bone Joint Surg Am 1985;67(1):1–7.

[59] Evans DL. Recurrent instability of the ankle; a method of surgical treatment. Proc R Soc Med 1953;46(5):343–4.

[60] van der Rijt AJ, Evans GA. The long-term results of Watson-Jones tenodesis. J Bone Joint Surg Br 1984;66(3):371–5.

[61] Anderson ME. Reconstruction of the lateral ligaments of the ankle using the plantaris tendon. J Bone Joint Surg Am 1985;67(6):930–4.

[62] Segesser B, Goesele A. Weber fibular ligament-plasty with plantar tendon with Segesser modification. Sportverletz Sportschaden 1996;10(4):88–93.

[63] Harvey FJ, Chu G, Harvey PM. Surgical availability of the plantaris tendon. J Hand Surg Am 1983;8(3):243–7.

[64] Saxena A, Bareither D. Magnetic resonance and cadaveric findings of the incidence of plantaris tendon. Foot Ankle Int 2000;21(7):570–2.

[65] Daseler EH, Anson BH. The plantaris muscle. An anatomical study of 750 specimens. JBJS 1943;25:822–7.

[66] Tillmann B, Töndury G. Flexorengruppe der unteren Extremität. In: Leonhardt H, Tillmann B, Töndury G, Zilles K, editors. Bewegungsapparat. Stuttgart: Thieme; 1987. p. 584–793.

[67] Hintermann B, Holzach P, Matter P. The treatment of fibular ligament lesions using the Ortho-Rehab shoe. Schweiz Z Sportmed 1990;38(2):87–93.

[68] Magerl F, Marti R. Fibulotalar ligament replacement using the plantaris tendon. Hefte Unfallheilkd 1978;133:169–74.

[69] Krips R, van Dijk CN, Lehtonen H, et al. Sports activity level after surgical treatment for chronic anterolateral ankle instability. A multicenter study. Am J Sports Med 2002;30(1): 13–9.

[70] Krips R, van Dijk CN, Halasi T, et al. Anatomical reconstruction versus tenodesis for the treatment of chronic anterolateral instability of the ankle joint: a 2- to 10-year follow-up, multicenter study. Knee Surg Sports Traumatol Arthrosc 2000;8(3):173–9.

ELSEVIER
SAUNDERS

Foot Ankle Clin N Am
11 (2006) 585–595

**FOOT AND
ANKLE CLINICS**

Anatomic Reconstruction of the Lateral Ligament Complex of the Ankle Using a Gracilis Autograft

Dory S. Boyer, MD, FRCSC,
Alastair S.E. Younger, MB ChB, ChM, MSc, FRCSC*

*British Columbia's Foot and Ankle Clinic, Suite 560 1144 Burrard Street, Vancouver,
British Columbia, Canada V6Z 3E8*

Injuries to the lateral ligament complex of the ankle injuries are common in recreational and competitive athletes [1]. Most resolve with little medical intervention, and recurrent instability occurs in 15% to 48% of these injuries [2–6]. After nonoperative management, including physiotherapy and bracing, continued problems may require surgical intervention. Reestablishing ankle stability and proper biomechanics may be important to prevent osteoarthritis [7,8].

Many procedures are available for the management for lateral ankle instability [2,7,9–11], with an overall success for correction of instability greater than 80% [12]. There is little evidence that one procedure is preferable to others, and one can group the procedures into three categories: anatomic repair, nonanatomic reconstruction, and anatomic reconstruction.

Anatomic repairs are the most straightforward, and involve using the injured ligaments to reconstitute the new lateral stabilizing complex, with a success rate of 88% to 95% [13,14]. The Brostrom procedure with a Gould modification [15,16] uses the remaining anterior talo-fibular ligament (ATFL) and calcaneofibular ligament (CFL) tissue augmented by local extensor retinaculum [14], allowing restoration of stability [13,16].

The use of anatomic repairs is limited to patients with local tissues durable enough for repair [17]. Recurrent ankle sprains and multiple previous procedures will often leave patulous local tissues insufficient to perform their role as a restraint to inversion internal rotation. Suture anchors help augment the repair [18]. Contraindications to anatomic repair may include

* Corresponding author.
E-mail address: asyounger@shaw.ca (A.S.E. Younger).

1083-7515/06/$ - see front matter © 2006 Elsevier Inc. All rights reserved.
doi:10.1016/j.fcl.2006.06.017
foot.theclinics.com

long-standing ankle instability, high athletics patient demands, second-attempt surgery, generalized ligamentous laxity, as well as unfavorable patient habitus [6,19,20]. An ATFL repair in isolation, may not limit pathologic subtalar motion.

Nonanatomic reconstructions will improve stability in the ankle, but without documented improved outcomes over anatomic repairs. These reconstructions involve replacing the lateral ligament complex with a tenodesis using tissue autograft. Favorable short-term results with this type of reconstruction have been demonstrated, but tibiotalar osteoarthritis with long-term follow-up has been observered [21]. The Crisman-Snook, Evans, and Watson-Jones tenodesis procedures require the harvesting the peroneus brevis tendon, either whole or in part [9,22]. The only one uniquely stabilizing the subtalar joint is the Chrisman-Snook prodedure [23]. Persistent instability impairs up to 19% of these ankles [24]. Decreased range of motion and a low rate of return to full activities affect nonanatomic reconstructions [25]. Return rates to full activity can be only 52% [26].

Biomechanical overdrive of the peroneus longus and decreased ankle eversion strength are direct sequelae of harvesting the peroneus brevis tendon. In chronic instability, the peroneus longus tendon may also be damaged or impaired [21]. Dynamic stabilization of the ankle may be lost using the tendon of peroneus brevis. A nonanatomic reconstruction, while reducing subtalar motion, does not restore proper ankle mechanics [27]. In the short term, this manifests as stiffness, but longitudinal studies demonstrated tibiotalar osteoarthritis in 19% to 28% of patients [2,28]. Also, subjective complaints of stiffness following reconstruction are common, albeit without subjective dissatisfaction with the procedure [2,29]. Loss of motion follows nonanatomic reconstruction [30,31], and this may be associated with chronic ankle and subtalar osteoarthritis [32]. The results of nonanatomic reconstruction generally deteriorate with time [2,33,34].

Anatomic reconstruction using various graft choices produce lower rates of recurrent instability with improved patient outcomes over nonanatomic reconstruction [35]. Most procedures are a modification of the original description of Elmslie. These procedures anatomically reconstruct the severed or torn ligaments using the normal tissues as a guide. This would ideally control anterior translation and rotational stability while preserving proper joint biomechanics [2]. Coupled with restoration of normal ankle and foot biomechanics, recurrence rates for instability ranged from 0% to 3% [36], with good/excellent outcomes in 91% to 100% of patients [6,37].

Choices for grafts have included semitendinosus [10], gracilis [6,38], plantaris, palmaris [37], fascia lata, bone–patellar tendon [39], and allografts. The mechanical properties of autografts are generally superior to those of the repaired ligaments. Graft choice must take into account any associated harvest site morbidity. Artificial ligaments have been described with uncertain long-term effects [40]. We prefer the use of the gracilis tendon, as its use in a four-strand hamstring anterior cruciate ligament repair demonstrates minimal donor site morbidity. Anatomic reconstruction using the gracilis was first described in 2001 [6,38]. However, Coughlin's method of tendon attatchment is different, as outlined in the rest of the article. Choice of this autogenous graft has many advantages. Its strength and lack of associated morbidity is well known. The most common complaint after using this graft is mild anesthesia secondary to saphenous nerve irritation. Preservation of the semitendinosus tendon will reduce hamstring weakness noted following anterior cruciate ligament reconstruction. Also, the harvest site is within the surgical field under tourniquet control, and requires little time for harvest.

An ideal procedure restores normal ankle motion and stability while maintaining proper hindfoot biomechanics. A swift and uncomplicated return to activities without the late sequelae of stiffness and osteoarthritis are also ideal.

Surgical technique

After general anesthesia in induced, a well-padded wide-thigh tourniquet is placed. The hip on the operative side is elevated to allow for lateral exposure. A careful examination under anesthesia is performed, focusing on side-to-side comparison. Often, this can be quite different from a clinical office examination, and is more reliable than preoperative talar tilt assessment.

Preoperative antibiotics are administered as dictated by hospital protocol. Sterile prepping and draping of the patient are performed, and the limb is exsanguinated using gravity. A five-nerve ankle block is used.

Diagnostic ankle arthroscopy is first performed and a standard 21-point inspection is accomplished. The intraarticular pathologies associated with lateral ligament injuries include osteochondral defects on the talus and tibia, synovitis, and loose bodies [41,42]. These are documented and addressed. Medial deltoid ligament injuries are also seen in conjuction with lateral instability [43]. Arthroscopic examination can assist in the diagnosis. After addressing any intraarticular pathology, the scope is withdrawn and the soft tissues squeezed to allow for extravasation of any excess fluid.

A curvilinear incision is made parallel to and just anterior to the posterior border of the fibula, curving anteriorly, ending just proximal to the calcaneocuboid joint (Fig. 1). The soft tissues are carefully dissected, and crossing branches of the superficial peroneal and sural nerves are identified and protected. The ankle joint is approached after division of the extensor retinaculum and following the extensor tendons to the level of the ankle joint. The capsule is entered at the junction of the tibia, talus, and fibula. The anterior talofibular ligament is identified and kept intact. The anterolateral aspect of the talus is exposed. At this point, an open anterior drawer inversion stress examination is performed, demonstrating any pathologic laxity within the anterior talofibular ligament (Fig. 2). This is our standard for the diagnosis of pathologic ATFL insufficiency.

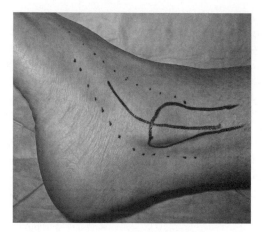

Fig. 1. Incisions required for the procedure.

The peroneal retinaculum is incised, exposing the tendons of peroneus brevis and peroneus longus. They are examined for any tears or synovial hypertrophy, as both conditions can be associated with chronic lateral ankle instability. Varus and valgus motions of the foot allow for a large expanse of the tendon to be seen and palpated under direct vision. The calcaneofibular ligament is located on the floor of the tunnel and isolated. Subtalar motion is assessed with the CFL directly visible.

If only one ligament is damaged, an anatomic repair of the isolated ligament is performed using the Brostom procedure with a Gould modification. If both ligaments are torn, the talus is exposed toward the neck, allowing for

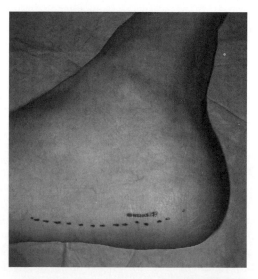

Fig. 2. Incisions required for the procedure.

the future entry point of a fixation screw. The ATFL and the CFL and transected producing fresh ligament edges and delineating the anatomy of the distal fibula, allowing for anatomic reconstruction of the lateral restraints using our tendon weave.

The gracilis tendon is then harvested using a 1 to 1.5-cm incision over the insertion of the ipsilateral pes anserinus. Careful dissection down to the level of the sartorial fascia reduces the possibility of saphenous nerve injury. A tendon stripper is employed for gracilis harvest, maintaining the tendon insertion distally. After the muscle is removed using a ribboncurl motion with mayo scissors, a #2 Ethibond suture is woven into the end of the tendon using a running, locking weave. The distal insertion is removed, preserving as much of the voluminous, thick tendon end. The tendon is then placed in a moist sponge to prevent drying out.

A 1-cm incision is made over the medial aspect of the calcaneal body with careful spreading to the bone (Fig. 1). The location of this incision is directly adjacent to the Achilles insertion with its dense fascia, sufficiently distal and posterior to the tip of the malleolus to avoid any complications that may arise by interrupting any of the neurovascular structures that course posterior to it. Depending on the tendon size, a 4.5-mm or 6-mm drill is used through this incision to produce a tunnel that runs to the CFL insertion on the calcaneus.

A 4.5-mm or 6-mm drill is used to create the tunnels on the distal fibula (Fig. 3). The first entry point for the drill is at the origin of the CFL, exiting through the posterior cortex, allowing for a bony bridge. The second passage of the drill is from the ATFL origin posteriorly, about 1 cm proximal to the initial exiting drill hole in the fibula. Great care must be taken to preserve

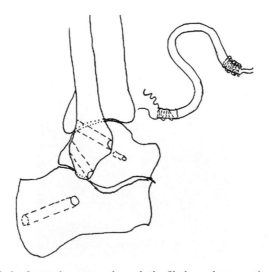

Fig. 3. Drill holes for tendon weave through the fibula, and preparation of the graft.

the integrity of the fibular cortex; otherwise, an effective tendon weave will be very difficult to achieve. Also, the peroneal tendons must be retracted so that further damage is avoided to them from any contact with the drill bit.

Returning to the medial incision, the fibrous end of the gracilis (distal harvest) is sutured into the medial border of the Achilles tendon insertion adjacent to the drill tunnel. The tendon is passed using a suture passer with weaved end going through the calcaneus (Fig. 4). The fibrous end of the graft is allowed to pass into the tunnel where it is anchored using a #2 Ethibond suture. Allowing the graft end to enter the tunnel avoids any buildup of suture and ligament that could cause subcutaneous irritation medially.

The surgeon should position the hindfoot carefully when the graft is secured. Eversion of the hindfoot is essential. The tendon is taken through the posterior fibular tunnel (CFL origin) and then back through the second fibular tunnel (out the ATFL origin) (Fig. 5). Further securing of the graft is undertaken at each step with the #1 Vicryl to the periosteum. A small fragment 3.5-mm cancellous screw with a small and large fragment washer are inserted into the lateral talus at the site of the ATFL insertion (Fig. 6). The graft is passed under the screw on the right ankle, and over the screw on the left, so that the graft is tensioned as the screw is tightened with the ankle in dorsiflexion. The tendon is then sewn onto itself offering a more robust ATFL substance. If the graft is long enough, the end is sutured back onto the periosteum of the fibula. We avoid the use of a drill hole in the talar neck, as this may cause a stress riser and risk fracture (Fig. 7).

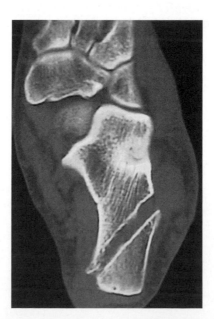

Fig. 4. CT scan delineating the course of the calcaneal tunnel.

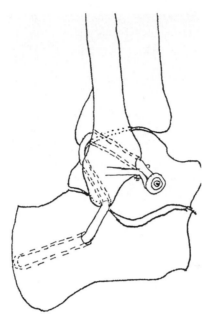

Fig. 5. Drawing of lateral ankle demonstrating the overall course of the gracilis tendon.

With the graft secure, the peroneal retinaculum is sutured following any tendon repair that might be indicated. The stability of the medial ligament complex is then examined by an anterior drawer while feeling for translation within the medial ankle from the lateral wound. The presence of medial ligament instability with lateral ligament instability is well documented, and repairs to this complex may also be necessary.

Additional procedures such as a calcaneal osteotomy, gastrocnemius slide, or peroneal tendon augmentation with a tendon transfer may also be indicated.

The wounds are copiously irrigated, and the tourniquet released to facilitate hemostasis. Skin closure is finished with a running 3-0 Nylon, and the limb is protected with a well-padded nonweight bearing short-leg splint.

Rehabilitation protocol

We allow patients to fully weight bear after 2 weeks following surgery, coinciding with the removal of the plaster splint. This allows ample time for healing of the skin wound. Sutures are removed at this time, and the patient is placed into a walker boot for comfort. Removal of the boot is permitted for range of motion up to four times per day. We begin physiotherapy as soon as the postoperative splint is removed to facilitate edema control, and educate the patient regarding the movements permitted.

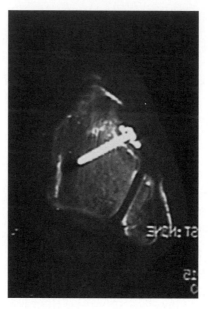

Fig. 6. CT scan delineating the position of the talar screw.

Placement in the walker boot prevents ankle inversion while the tendon incorporates into the bony tunnels. Stationary bicycling is begun after 4 weeks, and the walker boot is discontinued after 10 weeks. The patient may return to full activities after 12 weeks.

While performing the accelerated rehab protocol, we recommend use of a brace exerting circumferential ankle pressure to help improve proprioceptive feedback.

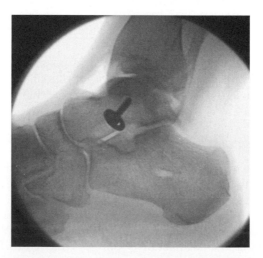

Fig. 7. Radiographs of screw position in the talus.

Outcomes

Ideally, a reconstructive procedure should restore normal ankle motion and stability while maintaining proper hindfoot biomechanics, allowing for a swift and uncomplicated return to activities without the late sequellae of stiffness and osteoarthritis. Any surgical procedure aimed at recreating proper lateral ankle retraints must be accompanied by deformity correction or the instability may recur.

For atheletes with increased focus on loss of playing time and more functional recovery, an aggressive rehabilitation protocol allowing earlier return to activity provides an overall functional recovery of the ankle. Procedures using anatomic reconstruction can facilitate this earlier return to activity. Anatomic repair procedures usually necessitate a 6-week course of immobilization, and casting may result in unwanted postoperative stiffness, deconditioning of other lower extremity muscles, favoring this alternate approach.

We performed a cadaver study using the gracilis tendon reconstruction in comparison to a Brostrom repair. Comparisons were made as to the ability to restore adequate lateral ankle constraints as well as loss of range of motion. Seven cadaver ankles were tested sequentially intact, following lateral ligament resection, post-Brostom repair, and finally, postgracilis reconstruction. The study indicates a stronger initial repair occurs in the anatomic reconstruction, and range of motion is preserved in the ankle (unpublished data).

Summary

Many techniques have been described for surgical management of lateral ankle instability. Anatomic repair and nonanatomic reconstruction have higher recurrence rates, and may be complicated by ankle stiffness. Anatomic reconstruction should be considered in stabilization for deficiencies of the lateral ankle ligament complex, as the initial construct is stronger while maintaining normal ankle mechanics.

The gracilis autograft is a substantial graft that can be used safely to accomplish these goals with minimal patient morbidity. Our technique offers equivalent stability to a native ligament complex without decreasing range of motion and disrupting normal ankle mechanics. Early range of motion may be used for a quicker return to activities.

Further study of this type of anatomic reconstruction will be required to determine long term outcomes.

References

[1] Mack RP. Ankle injuries in athletics. Clin Sports Med 1982;1(1):71–84.
[2] Sammarco VJ. Complications of lateral ankle ligament reconstruction. Clin Orthop Relat Res 2001;391:123–32.

 [3] Bosien WR, Staples OS, Russell SW. Residual disability following acute ankle sprains. J Bone Joint Surg Am 1955;37-A(6):1237–43.
 [4] Brostrom L. Sprained ankles. V. Treatment and prognosis in recent ligament ruptures. Acta Chir Scand 1966;132(5):537–50.
 [5] Freeman MA. Instability of the foot after injuries to the lateral ligament of the ankle. J Bone Joint Surg Br 1965;47(4):669–77.
 [6] Coughlin MJ, Schenck RC Jr, Grebing BR, et al. Comprehensive reconstruction of the lateral ankle for chronic instability using a free gracilis graft. Foot Ankle Int 2004;25(4):231–41.
 [7] Harrington KD. Degenerative arthritis of the ankle secondary to long-standing lateral ligament instability. J Bone Joint Surg Am 1979;61(3):354–61.
 [8] Gross P, Marti B. Risk of degenerative ankle joint disease in volleball players. Study of former elite atheletes. Int J Sports Med 1999;20(1):58–63.
 [9] Evans DL. Recurrent instability of the ankle; a method of surgical treatment. Proc R Soc Med 1953;46(5):343–4.
[10] Paterson R, Cohen B, Taylor D, et al. Reconstruction of the lateral ligaments of the ankle using semi-tendinosis graft. Foot Ankle Int 2000;21(5):413–9.
[11] Peters JW, Trevino SG, Renstrom PA. Chronic lateral ankle instability. Foot Ankle 1991; 12(3):182–91.
[12] Colville MR. Surgical treatment of the unstable ankle. J Am Acad Orthop Surg 1998;6(6): 368–77.
[13] Liu SH, Jacobson KE. A new operation for chronic lateral ankle instability. J Bone Joint Surg Br 1995;77(1):55–9.
[14] Chen CY, Huang PJ, Kao KF, et al. Surgical reconstruction for chronic lateral instability of the ankle. Injury 2004;35(8):809–13.
[15] Gould N, Seligson D, Gassman J. Early and late repair of lateral ligament of the ankle. Foot Ankle 1980;1(2):84–9.
[16] Hamilton WG, Thompson FM, Snow SW. The modified Brostrom procedure for lateral ankle instability. Foot Ankle 1993;14(1):1–7.
[17] Barbari S, Brevig K, Egge T. Reconstruction of the lateral ligamentous structures of the ankle with a modified Watson-Jones procedure. Foot Ankle 1987;7(6):362–8.
[18] Paden MH, Stone PA, McGarry JJ. Modified Brostrom lateral ankle stabilization utilizing an implantable anchoring system. J Foot Ankle Surg 1994;33(6):617–22.
[19] Girard P, Anderson RB, Davis WH, et al. Clinical evaluation of the modified Brostrom-Evans procedure to restore ankle stability. Foot Ankle Int 1999;20(4):246–52.
[20] Karlsson J, Lansinger O. Chronic lateral instability of the ankle in athletes. Sports Med 1993; 16(5):355–65.
[21] Rosenbaum D, Becker H, Sterk J, et al. Functional evaluation of the 10 year outcome after modified Evans repair for chronic ankle instability. Foot Ankle Int 1997;18:765–71.
[22] Snook G, Chrisman O, Wilson T. Long-term results of the Chrisman-Snook operation for reconstruction of the lateral ligaments of the ankle. J Bone Joint Surg Am 1985;67(1):1–7.
[23] Smith P, Miller S, Berni A. A modified Christman-Snook procedure for reconstruction of the lateral ligaments of the ankle: review of 18 cases. Foot Ankle Int 1995;16(5):259–66.
[24] Hennrikus W, Mapes R, Lyons P, et al. Outcomes of the Christman-Snook and modified Brostrom procedures for chronic lateral ankle instability: a prospective randomized comparison. Am J Sports Med 1996;24(4):400–4.
[25] Letts M, Davidson D, Mukhtar I. Surgical management of chronic lateral ankle instability in adolescents. J Pediatr Orthop 2003;23(3):392–7.
[26] Kaikkonen A, Hyppanen E, Kannus P, et al. Long-term functional outcome after primary repair of the lateral ligaments of the ankle. Am J Sports Med 1997;25(2):150–5.
[27] Colville MR, Marder RA, Zarins B. Reconstruction of the lateral ankle ligaments. A biomechanical analysis. Am J Sports Med 1992;20(5):594–600.
[28] Becker HP, Rosenbaum D. Chronic recurrent ligament instability on the lateral ankle. Orthopade 1999;28(6):483–92.

[29] Hoy K, Lindblad BE, Terkelsen CJ, et al. Badminton injuries—a prospective epidemiological and socioeconomic study. Br J Sports Med 1994;28(4):276–9.

[30] Kaikkonen A, Lehtonen H, Kannus P, et al. Long term functional outcome after surgery of chronic ankle instability: a 5-year follow-up study of the modified Evans procedure. Scand J Med Sci Sports 1999;9(4):239–44.

[31] Baltopoulos P, Tzagarakis G, Kaseta M. Midterm results of a modified Evans repair for chronic lateral ankle instability. Clin Orthop 2004;422:180–5.

[32] Schmidt R, Cordier E, Bertsch C, et al. Reconstruction of the lateral ligaments: do the anatomic procedures restore physiologic ankle kinematics? Foot Ankle Int 2004;25:31–6.

[33] Karlsson J, Brandsson S, Kalebo P, et al. Surgical treatment of concomitant chronic ankle instability and longitudinal rupture of the peroneus brevis tendon. Scand J Med Sci Sports 1998;8(1):42–9.

[34] Hintermann B. Biomechanics of the ligaments of the unstable ankle joint. Sportverletz Sportschaden 1996;10(3):48–54.

[35] Kripps R, van Dijk C, Lehtonen H, et al. Sports activity level after surgical treatment for chronic anterolateral ankle instability. A multicenter study. Am J Sports Med 2002;30:13–9.

[36] Sammarco GJ, DiRaimondo CV. Surgical treatment of lateral ankle instability syndrome. Am J Sports Med 1988;16(5):501–11.

[37] Okuda R, Kinoshita M, Morikawa J, et al. Reconstruction for chronic lateral ankle instability using the palmaris longus tendon: is reconstruction of the calcaneofibular ligament neccessary? Foot Ankle Int 1999;20(11):714–20.

[38] Coughlin MJ, Matt V, Schenck RC Jr. Augmented lateral ankle reconstruction using a free gracilis graft. Orthopedics 2002;25(1):31–5.

[39] Sugimoto K, Takakura Y, Kumai T, et al. Reconstruction of the lateral ankle ligaments with bone patellar bone tendon graft in patients with chronic ankle instability: A preliminary report. Am J Sports Med 2002;30:340–6.

[40] Usami N, Inokuchi S, Hiraishi E, et al. Clinical application of artificial ligament for ankle instability—long term follow up. J Long Term Eff Med Implants 2000;10(4):239–50.

[41] Komenda GA, Ferkel RD. Arthroscopic findings associated with the unstable ankle. Foot Ankle Int 1999;20(11):708–13.

[42] Okuda R, Kinoshita M, Morikawa J, et al. Arthroscopic findings in chronic lateral ankle instability: do focal chondral lesions influence the results of ligament reconsrtruction? Am J Sports Med 2005;33:35–42.

[43] Hintermann B, Boss A, Schafer D. Arthroscopic findings in patients with chronic ankle instability. Am J Sports Med 2002;30(3):402–9.

ELSEVIER
SAUNDERS

Foot Ankle Clin N Am
11 (2006) 597–605

FOOT AND
ANKLE CLINICS

Reconstruction of the Lateral Ankle Ligaments with Allograft in Patients with Chronic Ankle Instability

Alessandro Caprio, MD[a],
Francesco Oliva, MD[b], Fabio Treia, MD[c],
Nicola Maffulli, MD, MS, PhD, FRCS (Orth)[d],*

[a]Paideia Hospital, Orthopaedic Unit, Via Vincenzo Tiberio 46, Rome, Italy
[b]University of Rome Tor Vergata, Faculty of Medicine and Surgery, Department of
Orthopaedics and Traumatology, Viale Oxford 81, 00133 Rome, Italy
[c]S. Luca Hospital, Orthopaedic Unit, Via Teano 8 A, Rome, Italy
[d]Department of Trauma and Orthopaedic Surgery, Keele University School of Medicine,
North Staffordshire Hospital, Thornburrow Drive, Hartshill, Stoke on Trent, Staffordshire,
ST4 7QB, United Kingdom

Fifteen percent to 25% of all injuries to the human musculoskeletal system are sprains of the lateral ankle ligaments [1]. In the United Kingdom, the crude incidence rate of ankle sprains was 52.7 per 10 000 of accident and emergency attendances, rising to 60.9 (95% confidence interval 59.4 to 62.4) when adjusted for the proportion of patients without a diagnostic code (13.7%) [2]. Functional rehabilitation can achieve excellent results in 70% to 85% of all grades of ankle sprain [3]. Twenty percent to 40% of patients with severe sprains will have continued pain and instability [4]. The lateral ligamentous complex of the ankle consists of the anterior talofibular ligament (ATFL), the calcaneofibular ligament (CFL), and the posterior talofibular ligament (PTFL). The lateral talocalcaneal ligament (LTCL) may or may not be present. When present, it limits subtalar motion [5,6].

The ATFL is the primary restraint to inversion of the ankle throughout its arc of motion. Strain to the ATFL increases progressively as the ankle moves into plantar flexion and inversion. As a result, the ATFL is usually torn in inversion, plantar flexion, and internal rotation. The CFL stabilizes both the ankle and the subtalar joints. Strain to the CFL is greatest when the

* Corresponding author.
  E-mail address: n.maffulli@keele.ac.uk (N. Maffulli).

1083-7515/06/$ - see front matter © 2006 Elsevier Inc. All rights reserved.
doi:10.1016/j.fcl.2006.05.003

ankle is inverted and dorsiflexed. The CFL tears primarily in inversion and ankle dorsiflexion. The PTFL is rarely injured unless complete dislocation occurs [7].

At operation, Brostrom [8] found that all patients with recurrent inversion instability had a tear of the ATFL. He also found that 27% of his 60 patients also had an injury to the CFL. More recently, a higher rate of combined injuries to the ATFL and the CFL has been demonstrated [9–11]. Although lesions of the ATFL must be addressed in all patients, most will also need reconstruction of the CFL to regain stability of both the ankle and the subtalar joints, and to avoid recurrence [12]. Although most patients do well with a Brostrom-type anatomic ligament repair, there remains a subset of patients who continue to experience recurrent instability.

The optimal management of chronic lateral ankle instability is controversial. Many surgical procedures have been recommended with variable success. Reconstruction using one of the peroneal tendons, most often peroneus brevis, is commonly performed [13–17], but restoration of normal mechanical restraints is not achieved with these procedures, as they act mainly as tenodeses [18,19]. The anatomic repair of the lateral ligaments originally described by Bostrom [8] was later modified by Gould [20]. End-to-end repair of the ruptured ligaments is possible even several years after the initial injury [8], but healing with intervening scar tissue or lengthening caused insufficiency [21]. The ideal reconstruction should restore the natural or original anatomy. Many of the reconstruction procedures sacrifice normal tissue, and the reconstructed ligaments are far from anatomic, altering the kinematics and resulting in limited joint motion, which may later cause degenerative joint disease [22].

Allograft tissues have several advantages, including shorter operative time, better cosmesis, availability of larger grafts, lower incidence of postoperative arthrofibrosis, reduced postoperative pain, and postoperative complications. Additionally, allografts provide a graft source when autogenic sources are not available or appropriate and, most important, no donor site morbidity. However, disadvantages of allografts include the risk of disease transmission, possibly slower incorporation rate in animal models, the potential for a subclinical immune response, and increased cost [23].

We describe an augmented reconstruction technique of ATFL and CFL reconstruction with a semitendinosus tendon allograft through a peroneal bone tunnel fixed with biodegradable anchors.

Preoperative planning

The assessment of instability is made clinically. A comprehensive examination of the ankle and foot is required to assess these structures and to exclude other pathology. We do not routinely perform radiographic stress tests: there are insufficient data for comparison of the use of mechanical versus manual techniques, and they document laxity, not instability [24].

As initial acute ankle sprains are initially managed in a functional nonoperative fashion, and as management does not depend on the degree of ankle laxity on stress views, but on subjective instability, the talar tilt and anterior drawer stress radiographs have no clinical relevance in the acute situation. In patients with chronic instability, the large variability in talar tilt and anterior drawer values in both injured and noninjured ankles precludes their routine use [24].

Operative technique

The procedure is performed under general anesthetic. A diagnostic ankle arthroscopy is routinely made.

Graft preparation

We used a commercially available allogeneic semitendinosus tendon graft cryopreserved at −80°C (Careggi Civil Hospital, Bone Bank Department, Florence, Italy). The graft was reconstituted in sterile saline with 1 g of Cefamandole (Cefamandolo, Mandokef, Eli Lilly SpA, Rome, Italy) for 15 minutes at 40°. We tested the allograft for Gram-positive and -negative microorganisms. Two nonabsorbable #1 vicryl (Ethicon, Edinburgh, UK) sutures were placed at each end in a running fashion.

Position

The patient is placed supine on the operating table with a sandbag under the buttock of the operative side to internally rotate the affected leg.

Antibiotic prophylaxis

A single dose of a first generation cephalosporin is administered at induction of anesthesia.

Tourniquet

The limb to be operated on is exsanguinated, and a tourniquet on the thigh of the injured leg is inflated to 250 mmHg.

Incision

A 4-cm to 6-cm incision is made centered on the lateral malleolus toward the base of the fifth metatarsal with the foot held in plantarflexion.

Procedure

In the distal part of the incision, the sinus tarsi of the subtalar joint is opened, and scar tissue is debrided, as it is often a source of pain. The subcutaneous tissues are exposed. If healthy margins of the ATFL and CFL are seen, a modified Broström procedure is performed. After thorough evaluation of these two ligaments, a 1.6-mm Kirschner wire is drilled from anterosuperior to posteroinferior at an angle of 25° between the Kirschner wire and a horizontal line passing through to the tip of the distal fibula. A tunnel 4.5 mm in diameter is drilled (Fig. 1a and b). The semitendinosus allograft is passed through this tunnel (Fig. 2a and b). The correct insertion point is identified by dissecting and identifying the torn or attenuated ligament, and tracing it to its attachment point on the calcaneus and talus, respectively. The neo ATFL and CFL are placed in their anatomic position at an angulation between 80° and 130°, and accurately sutured with vycril 2/0 (Ethicon, Edinburgh, UK) to the periosteum at the entrance and exit holes tunnels. The portion of the allograft used for to reconstruction the CFL should be routed underneath the peroneals (Fig. 3).

With the ankle held in neutral dorsiflexion and plantarflexion and neutral inversion and eversion, the allograft is anchored to the talus and the calcaneus with bioassorbable anchors (Spiraloc Mitek Products, Inc., Norwood, Massachusetts) tensioning the allograft by hand. The wounds are closed in layers with 2/0 vicryl (Ethicon, Edinburgh, UK), an undyed 3/0 vicryl (Ethicon, Edinburgh, UK) subcuticular suture and steristrips (3M, Loughborough, UK).

A nonadherent dressing, velband and crepe bandage are applied. A below-knee walking synthetic cast is applied with the ankle in neutral position.

Postoperative management

No weight bearing is allowed for 2 weeks, when the plaster is removed. The patient is placed into a removable walking boot locked at neutral

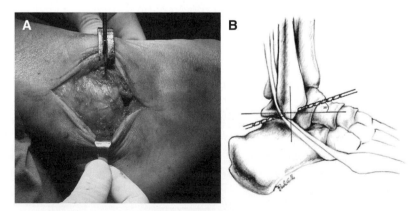

Fig. 1. (*A*) A Kirschner wire is drilled from anterosuperior to posteroinferior at an angle of 25° between the Kirschner wire and a line parallel to the tip of the distal fibula. (*B*) A tunnel 4.5 mm in diameter is drilled.

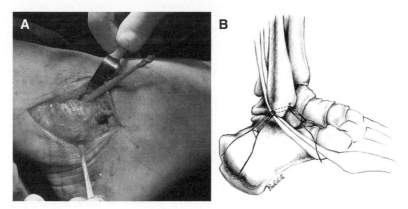

Fig. 2. (*A*) The semitendinosus allograft is passed through the peroneal tunnel. (*B*) The graft is accurately sutured with vycril 2/0 to the periosteum at the entrance and exit holes of the peroneal tunnel.

(Donjoy MC Walker Donjoy Ro + Ten, Italy) for 4 weeks. Patients discard the boot three to four times a day to work on ankle dorsiflexion and plantarflexion. Partial weight bearing may begin at 2 weeks, progressing to full weight bearing by 4 weeks. Gentle active inversion and eversion may begin 4 weeks postoperatively, wobble board exercises. Bicycle training begins at 4 weeks in the boot. Six weeks postoperatively the boot is removed, and the patient is placed into an ankle stirrup brace full time for 4 weeks. Isometric exercises, heel raises, peroneal strength training, proprioceptive training, and balance exercises are begun at 6 weeks. Running, jumping, and sports-specific exercises are begun between 12 and 14 weeks based on the amount of swelling, and progress with earlier therapy goals. Use of the ankle brace during sports is encouraged for the next 6 to 9 months [25].

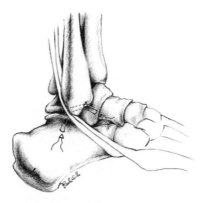

Fig. 3. The neo ATFL and CFL are placed in their anatomic position at an angle between 80° and 130°. The neo CFL must be routed underneath the peroneals. Two anchors are positioned in the anatomic insertion of the ATFL and CFL insertion.

Results

Between January 2003 and May 2004, 11 patients (8 males; 3 females) underwent reconstruction of the lateral ankle ligament complex with allograft using the above technique. Chronic lateral ankle instability and a failed trial of conservative treatment (protected mobilization and formal physical therapy) were the inclusion criteria. Patients were assessed prospectively with the modified American Orthopaedic Foot and Ankle Society (AOFAS) hindfoot score, physical examination, radiographs, and, when indicated, MRI. The AOFAS hindfoot scores improved significantly: Scores averaged 29.6 points preoperatively (standard deviation [SD], 15.6 points) and improved to 55.4 points (SD, 13.6 points) at an average follow up of 14.1 months ($P < 0.001$). The SF-12 mental component did not change significantly ($P = 0.25$). The SF-12 physical component improved significantly from a preoperative mean of 35.6 points (SD, 9.14 points) to a postoperative mean of 49.3 points (SD, 8.7; $P < 0.001$). There has been no revisional surgery.

Complications

Our patients showed no immunologic rejection, disease transmission, or inflammatory foreign body reaction.

The future

Cryopreservation, the method used for our study, is a process of controlled-rate freezing with the extraction of cellular water by the use of cryoprotectant media, including dimethylsulfoxide, in a proprietary formula at 1°C per minute to −135°C. The grafts finally were stored in liquid nitrogen at −196°C. This process, normally used to preserve sperm and embryos, prevents cell death by altering water crystallization within cells during freezing. Ligament cell survival and collagen production after the freezing procedure were described in an animal model [26]. The risk of harvesting and processing tissues from a donor who is human immunodeficiency virus antigen positive and antibody negative is currently estimated to be less than one in 1.5 million [27,28]. Allografts should be obtained only from tissue banks certified with the criteria of the American Association of Tissue Banks, and the patient should be informed of the potential for disease transmission preoperatively. Another disadvantage of our technique is the high cost of allograft. At our institution, a semitendinosus tendon allograft costs about 396 Euro (US$ 496.32).

We have used allogeneic tendon grafts to reconstruct the ligament in an anatomic fashion. Immunogenic rejection and disease transmission are potential problems when an allogenic tendon is used [29–32]. The major antigens are present on the tenocytes, and antigenicity is decreased by cryopreservation [33].

In previous experimental studies, transplanted fresh-frozen allogeneic tendon revascularized, with invasion of mesenchymal cells followed by reorganization of the collagen fibers. There was no evidence of immunologic rejection [34–36].

In other techniques using allografts or autografts that preserve peroneal tendon function, more than one bone tunnel is drilled, and the graft is secured with a variety of different devices [37–40].

Burks and Morgan [6] found that the ATFL originates 1 cm proximal to the tip of the lateral malleolus. The ligament averages 7.2 mm in width and inserts into the talus just distal to the articular surface, 18 mm proximal to the subtalar joint. The ATFL is contiguous with the joint capsule and not easily defined in patients who have sustained recurrent ankle sprains and instability. The CFL originates adjacent to the ATFL, approximately 8 mm proximal to the tip of the fibula, and courses posterior and distal to the calcaneus. The CFL inserts onto the calcaneus 13 mm distal to the subtalar joint. The CFL ligament is an extracapsular ligament, and makes up the floor of the peroneal sheath. The ATFL and the CFL insert at a conjoined site, at the ventral aspect of the distal fibula. Therefore, one can argue that all routing procedures that use the tip of the fibula as the new insertion of the CFL are not anatomic, and do not reproduce the correct anatomy of the ligaments, with the potential consequence of altering the biomechanics of the subtalar and ankle joint [39].

Ozeki and colleagues [41] reported that the isometric points of the ATFL and CF ligaments at the fibular attachments are such that drill holes in the fibula for the ATFL and CFL should be placed very close together or that one drill hole should be used for both ligaments.

The technique described here avoids the possibility of complications arising from bone tunnels in the talus and the calcaneus, as we anchor the distal ends of the allograft with bioadsorbable anchors. Furthermore, this technique avoids local morbidity.

References

[1] Komenda GA, Ferkel RD. Arthroscopic findings associated with the unstable ankle. Foot Ankle Int 1999;20:708–13.
[2] Bridgman SA, Clement D, Downing A, et al. Population based epidemiology of ankle sprains attending accident and emergency units in the West Midlands of England, and a survey of UK practice for severe ankle sprains. Emerg Med J 2003;20:508–10.
[3] Kannus P, Renstrom P. Treatment for acute tears of the lateral ligaments of the ankle. Operation, cast, or early controlled mobilization. J Bone Joint Surg Am 1991;73:305–12.
[4] Sammarco VJ. Complications of lateral ankle ligament reconstruction. Clin Orthop 2001; 391:123–32.
[5] Kumai T, Takakura Y, Rufai A, et al. The functional anatomy of the human anterior talofibular ligament in relation to ankle sprains. J Anat 2002;200:457–65.
[6] Burks RT, Morgan J. Anatomy of the lateral ankle ligaments. Am J Sports Med 1994;22: 72–7.

[7] Colville MR, Marder RA, Boyle JJ, et al. Strain measurement in lateral ankle ligaments. Am J Sports Med 1990;18:196–200.

[8] Brostrom L, Sprained ankles V. Treatment and prognosis in recent ligament ruptures. Acta Chir Scand 1966;132:537–50.

[9] Meyer JM, Garcia J, Hoffmeyer P, et al. The subtalar sprain. A roentgenographic study. Clin Orthop 1988;226:169–73.

[10] Moller-Larsen F, Wethelund JO, Jurik AG, et al. Comparison of three different treatments for ruptured lateral ankle ligaments. Acta Orthop Scand 1988;59:564–6.

[11] Sugimoto K, Takakura Y, Samoto N, et al. Subtalar arthrography in recurrent instability of the ankle. Clin Orthop Relat Res 2002;394:169–76.

[12] Colville MR. Reconstruction of the lateral ankle ligaments. Instr Course Lect 1995;44: 341–8.

[13] Evans DL. Recurrent instability of the ankle—a method of surgical treatment. Proc R Soc Med 1953;46:343–4.

[14] Chrisman OD, Snook GA. Reconstruction of lateral ligament tears of the ankle. An experimental study and clinical evaluation of seven patients treated by a new modification of the Elmslie procedure. J Bone Joint Surg Am 1969;51:904–12.

[15] Zenni EJ Jr, Grefer M, Krieg JK, et al. Lateral ligamentous instability of the ankle: a method of surgical reconstruction by a modified Watson-Jones technique. Am J Sports Med 1977;5: 78–83.

[16] Hedeboe J, Johannsen A. Recurrent instability of the ankle joint. Surgical repair by the Watson-Jones method. Acta Orthop Scand 1979;50:337–40.

[17] Horstman JK, Kantor GS, Samuelson KM. Investigation of lateral ankle ligament reconstruction. Foot Ankle 1981;1:338–42.

[18] Becker HP, Rosenbaum D, Zeithammer G, et al. Gait pattern analysis after ankle ligament reconstruction (modified Evans procedure). Foot Ankle Int 1994;15:477–82.

[19] Rosenbaum D, Becker HP, Wilke HJ, et al. Tenodeses destroy the kinematic coupling of the ankle joint complex: a three-dimensional in vitro analysis of joint movement. J Bone Joint Surg 1998;80B:162–8.

[20] Gould N, Seligson D, Gassman J. Early and late repair of lateral ligament of the ankle. Foot Ankle 1980;1:84–9.

[21] Ahlgren O, Larsson S. Reconstruction for lateral ligament injuries of the ankle. J Bone Joint Surg 1989;71-B:300–3.

[22] Rosenbaum D, Bertsch C, Claes LE. Tenodeses do not fully restore ankle joint loading characteristics: a biomechanical in vitro investigation in the hind foot. Clin Biomech (Bristol) 1997;12:202–9.

[23] Indelli PF, Dillingham MF, Fanton GS, et al. Anterior cruciate ligament reconstruction using cryopreserved allografts. Clin Orthop 2004;420:268–75.

[24] Frost SC, Amendola A. Is stress radiography necessary in the diagnosis of acute or chronic ankle instability? Clin J Sport Med 1999;9:40–5.

[25] O'Shea KJ. Technique for biotenodesis screw fixation in tendon-enhanced ankle ligament reconstruction. Tech Foot Ankle Surg 2003;2:40–6.

[26] Frank C, Edwards P, McDonald D, et al. Viability of ligaments after freezing: an experimental study in a rabbit model. J Orthop Res 1988;6:95–102.

[27] Buck BE, Resnick L, Shah SM, et al. Human immunodeficiency virus cultured from bone. Implications for transplantation. Clin Orthop 1990;251:249–53.

[28] Buck BE, Malinin TI, Brown MD. Bone transplantation and human immunodeficiency virus. An estimate of risk of acquired immunodeficiency syndrome (AIDS). Clin Orthop 1989; 240:129–36.

[29] Olson EJ, Harner CD, Fu FH, et al. Clinical use of fresh, frozen soft tissue allografts. Orthopedics 1992;15:1225–32.

[30] Cartmell JS, Dunn MG. Development of cell-seeded patellar tendon allografts for anterior cruciate ligament reconstruction. Tissue Eng 2004;10:1065–75.

[31] Kainer MA, Linden JV, Whaley DN, et al. Clostridium infections associated with musculo-skeletal–tissue allografts. N Engl J Med 2004;17:2564–71.

[32] Barbour SA, King W. The safe and effective use of allograft tissue—an update. Am J Sports Med 2003;31:791–7.

[33] Minami A, Isbii S, Ogino T, et al. Effect of the immunological antigenicity of the allogeneic tendons on tendongrafting. Hand 1982;14:111–9.

[34] Shino K, Kawasaki T, Hirose H, et al. Replacement of the anterior cruciate ligament by an allogenic tendon graft: an experimental study in the dog. J Bone Joint Surg Br 1984;66: 672–81.

[35] Horibe S, Shino K, Nagano J, et al. Replacing the medial collateral ligament with an allogenic tendon graft. J Bone Joint Surg Br 1990;72:1044–9.

[36] Horibe S, Shino K, Taga I, et al. Reconstruction of lateral ligaments of the ankle with allogenic tendon grafts. J Bone Joint Surg Br 1991;73:802–5.

[37] Couglin MJ, Schenck RC Jr, Grebing BR, et al. Comprehensive reconstruction of the lateral ankle for chronic instability using a free gracilis graft. Foot Ankle Int 2004;25(4):231–41.

[38] Sugimoto K, Takakura Y, Kumai T, et al. Reconstruction of the lateral ankle ligaments with bone–patellar tendon graft in patients with chronic ankle instability: a preliminary report. Am J Sports Med 2002;30:340–6.

[39] Pagenstert GI, Valderrabano V, Hintermann B. Lateral ankle ligament reconstruction with free plantaris tendon graft. Tech Foot Ankle Surg 2005;4:104–12.

[40] Nakata K, Shino K, Horibe S, et al. Reconstruction of the lateral ligaments of the ankle using solvent-dried and gamma-irradiated allogeneic fascia lata. J Bone Joint Surg Br 2000;82: 579–82.

[41] Ozeki S, Yasuda K, Kaneda K, et al. Analysis of the isometry for reconstruction of the lateral ankle ligaments. J Jpn Soc Surg Foot 1990;11:98–102.

ELSEVIER
SAUNDERS

Foot Ankle Clin N Am
11 (2006) 607–623

FOOT AND
ANKLE CLINICS

Chronic Ankle Instability: Management of Chronic Lateral Ligamentous Dysfunction and the Varus Tibiotalar Joint

Donald J. McBride, FRCS, FRCS (Orth and Trauma)*,
Chandru Ramamurthy, MRCS, DOrtho

*Orthopaedic and Trauma Departments, University Hospital of North Staffordshire,
Princes Road, Stoke-on-Trent, Staffordshire St4 7LN, United Kingdom*

Ligament injuries in the ankle are very common, usually affecting the lateral side. Medial ligament injuries are usually associated with fractures of the ankle [1].

Acute injuries usually involve the anterior talofibular ligament (ATFL) (40%), the anterior talofibular and calcaneofibular ligaments (CFL) (58%), or with the posterior talofibular ligament (2%). Their management remains controversial, but current evidence suggests a better outcome in Grade III injuries with surgical management compared with functional treatment and a below-knee cast for pain, stability, and early return to work [2].

In patients with chronic insufficiency, either functional or structural, one usually has to address pain, instability, and any associated intraarticular pathology, which may be managed arthroscopically. One may prevent longer term osteoarthritis [3] and manage subtalar instability depending on the procedure chosen [4]. There is growing evidence that varus tilt of the tibial plafond or of the tibiotalar joint (Fig. 1) is important in the development of chronic lateral ligamentous dysfunction [5–8] but there remains an element of "chicken and egg" in the debate. Clearly, however, when considering surgery one should be aware of hindfoot deformity including varus and cavovarus, hypermobility, obesity, subtalar instability, neurologic disorders,

---

* Corresponding author.
E-mail address: donald.j.mcbride@btopenworld.com (D.J. McBride).

1083-7515/06/$ - see front matter © 2006 Elsevier Inc. All rights reserved.
doi:10.1016/j.fcl.2006.07.009

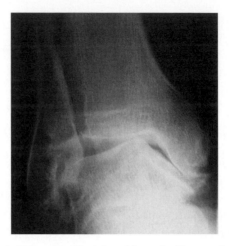

Fig. 1. Varus tibiotalar joint without significant arthritis.

intraarticular pathology, and of the so-called posterior fibula [9,10] or increased fibular mobility [11].

Basic anatomy and biomechanics

The lateral collateral ligament complex of the ankle is generally described, as a single functional unit comprised of three parts (Fig. 2). It is weaker and less extensive than the medial collateral ligament. The ATFL is attached laterally to the anterior border of the lateral malleolus, and passes anteromedially to the lateral surface of the neck of the talus. It blends partly with the ankle joint capsule, and is the weakest of the three

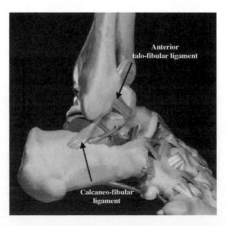

Fig. 2. Lateral ligamentous complex of the ankle joint.

components. The CFL lies deep to the peroneal tendons, and extends from the distal anterior border of the lateral malleolus inferiorly and posteriorly to attach to the upper part of the lateral surface of the os calcis. It is the largest of the three components. The strongest and deepest part is the posterior talofibular ligament, which is intracapsular but extrasynovial. It passes from its lateral attachment in the lower part of the lateral malleolar fossa to its medial attachment to the lateral tubercle of the posterior process of the talus. Other important ligaments include the anterior tibiofibular ligament, which extends obliquely distally and laterally from the anterior margin of the fibular notch of the tibia to the anterior border of the distal fibular shaft and lateral malleolus; the posterior tibiofibular ligament, which runs from the posterior surface of the lateral malleolus and upper part of the malleolar fossa of the fibula to the posterior aspect of the distal tibial shaft and posterior margin of the distal articular surface of the tibia; and the interosseous ligaments and membrane.

The bony anatomy includes the talus, tibia, and fibula, but there is an important relationship and link, in particular, with the subtalar joint and with the midfoot joints. Each bony and joint component is clearly stabilized by their congruence, the static and dynamic stabilizers, and by intact neuromuscular function.

Incidence and etiology

Acute lateral ligament injuries are common, comprising approximately 25% of all musculoskeletal injuries [12]. Approximately 5600 such injuries occur each day in the United Kingdom, approximately 23,000 occur each day in the United States, and 1600 in Holland [13,14]. What is less clear is the percentage of patients who will progress to develop chronic functional or structural instability; this may occur in 10% to 30% [15] or 10% to 20% [16]. The other main question relates to whether it is a condition waiting to happen similar to patellofemoral dysfunction.

There has been considerable research, particularly in the last decade, into the reasons why functional and structural chronic lateral instability develops in the ankle. Functional instability appears to have received the most attention. If one sets aside any anatomic considerations, then the previously healthy CFL tears primarily in inversion if the ankle is dorsiflexed; the ATFL tears in dorsiflexion, especially if combined with external rotation; and the posterior talofibular ligament tears with extreme dorsiflexion [17]. What happens thereafter may depend to some extent on management [2] and rehabilitation, but it is not clear what other factors contribute. The main problems appear to arise when there is impairment of neuromuscular coordination [18–21] and proprioceptive dysfunction [22–24], leading to gait abnormalities [25,26] and mechanical disturbance [27–29]. Current conservative and surgical management modalities discussed below should therefore be aimed at addressing these factors in the absence of any significant anatomic abnormality. However, the most important question still remains: Why does the ligament probably heal in most patients, but its supporting neurologic structures do not heal adequately in a substantial minority? The latter, of course, leads to greater risk of recurrent injury.

Turning to anatomic considerations, these have not received much attention until relatively recently. Varus or cavovarus deformity in the hindfoot, with or without neurologic dysfunction, may lead to lateral injury and dysfunction in the ankle [6,30] as may associated deformity elsewhere in the midfoot and forefoot [31]. Clearly, the integrity of the ligaments in individuals with hypermobility or endocrine syndromes or increased forces applied to the ligaments, for example, in obesity, are important. The roles of the posteriorly placed fibula [9,10] or increased mobility of the fibula [11] are being studied, and other factors may have to be considered, including the role of the anterolateral joint capsule [32], ossicles distinct from the lateral malleolus [33], and ununited osteochondral fractures of the distal fibula in adolescents [34].

Great interest currently is the location of the exact site of varus deformity in the hindfoot. In some patients, the deformity lies below the level of the ankle, usually in the os calcis and subtalar joint, and possibly, although not actually described, in the talus. A decrease in the anterior tip ratio (ATR) and its association with anterior drawer, particularly in female patients, has also been described [35]. This is a somewhat complicated measurement drawn from a lateral view of the ankle, and includes a perpendicular line with three tangential lines on the most proximal tibial surface, the most distal anterior tip of the tibia, and on the most distal posterior tip of the tibia (PTR). Points a, b, c, and d are determined on lines one and two for the ATR, with the anterior angle measured from a to b to c. The angle is small, and is made more meaningful by using the formula: ATR (%) = ab/ac × 100 = tan$A$ × 100. Sugimoto and colleagues [5] were the first to describe varus tilt of the tibial plafond as a factor in chronic ligament instability of the ankle. They studied 136 patients with acute ligament sprains and 85 patients with chronic lateral ligament instability, and measured varus angulation of the tibial plafond, varus angulation of the line passing through both malleolar ends, and varus angulation of the medial malleolus. The mean of each was larger in those patients with chronic ligament instability. McKinley and colleagues [36] investigated incongruity and instability in the etiology of posttraumatic arthritis using a dynamic ankle-testing device, and Valderrabano and colleagues [8] stated, "lateral ankle sprains in sports are the main cause of ligamentous posttraumatic ankle osteoarthritis and correlate with varus malalignment." They further concluded that persistent instability might still be present at the end stage of the disease process [8].

Clearly, in a significant proportion of patients both functional and anatomic features may be present. These may occur in both sedentary and athletic individuals. However, in the latter, there is a greater likelihood of exposure to injury, which may set the whole process off, particularly in adolescence.

Diagnosis

Diagnosis should normally be fairly straightforward in most acute lateral ligament sprains, taking care to confirm or refute any associated injuries, particularly osteochondral lesions. Management will depend on individual preference based on the current available evidence.

In chronic instability, due attention should be made to taking a thorough history, performing a thorough examination, and deciding on useful confirmatory tests. This process should be primarily aimed at differentiating between those patients who have developed osteoarthritis and might have associated deformity, and those who have not.

In most patients, the history is fairly consistent, with lateralized pain and swelling, particularly after an instability episode, recurrent instability sometimes over many years, and possibly many visits to a physiotherapist or orthotist in an attempt to stay away from a surgeon. The patient may have been or still is an avid sportsman, in the United Kingdom most frequently being labelled as having a "footballers ankle."

Examination will normally delineate tenderness with swelling, often over the anterolateral capsule or ligaments, with pain stressing the relevant ligaments affected. Some patients will have obvious laxity usually of the ATFL or CFL. An assessment should be made of ankle and subtalar motion in particular, but also of the joints of the midfoot and toes. Any hindfoot deformity, especially varus or cavovarus, should be noted. A Coleman Block test (Fig. 3) to confirm or refute fixed hindfoot deformity is helpful. A more general assessment should also be included, focusing specifically on obesity,

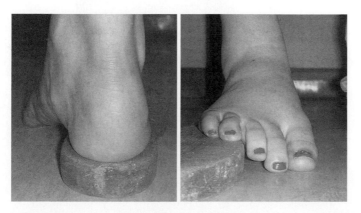

Fig. 3. Coleman block test.

hypermobility, endocrine disorders, neurologic disease, and circulatory impairment.

Confirmatory tests would normally include anteroposterior and lateral weight-bearing views of the ankle and foot, with anteroposterior and lateral comparative stress views (Fig. 4), although some doubt their reliability [37]. A Cobeys view or Brodens view may also be useful. Static ultrasound or MRI scans (Fig. 5) with or without arthrography [38] are not particularly helpful, but the latter may clarify other pathology [39], and dynamic assessment may be of use if personally supervised in selected patients. We do not routinely use arthrography [40]. However, a CT scan may help to clarify hindfoot varus deformity if surgical intervention is contemplated, so that this may be addressed [7]. We have a low threshold to proceeding to an examination under anesthesia or block with ankle arthroscopy [41,42]. We use this as part of the final diagnostic assessment and as a therapeutic device to manage a variety of associated conditions, including anterolateral impingement and synovitis and osteochondral lesions [43]. We also believe that it may be useful prognostically, and, in some patients, with preoperative agreement, more definitive surgery may be performed at the same sitting.

Management of chronic ligamentous dysfunction

Conservative management should be undertaken in all patients, even those in whom surgery is contemplated, as improving proprioception and muscular strength is important for postoperative rehabilitation. In a proportion of more sedentary patients with no sporting ambitions it may be all that is required. A further group may be happy with orthotics such as a lateral

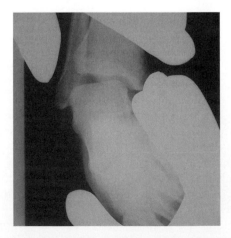

Fig. 4. Stress view of the ankle joint suggesting lateral ligamentous complex deficiency.

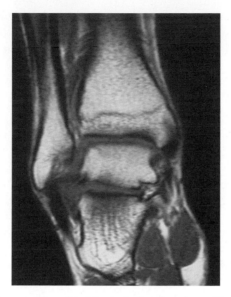

Fig. 5. MRI scan of the ankle joint including the calcaneofibular ligament.

wedge for the shoe or the variety of braces and supports currently available in addition to their rehabilitation program.

Surgery

The surgical group are likely to include athletes, either professional or amateur, dancers, those with marked instability either functional or structural, and those with osteoarthritis with or without deformity.

As far as ligamentous reconstruction is concerned, there are three broad groups:

1) anatomic repairs, for example, Brostrom [44], Brostrom-Gould [45], and their modifications;
2) periosteal substitution, for example, Rudert and colleagues [46];
3) peroneus brevis reconstruction, for example, Watson-Jones [47], Elmslie [48], Evans [49], Chrisman-Snook [50], and McBride and colleagues in press.

Several other procedures have been described recently that are not currently in routine use. These include bone–patellar tendon graft [51], pedicle tendon extensor hallucis longus (EHL) [52], transfer extensor digitorum brevis (EDB) [53], hamstring autograft [54], free gracilis graft [55], minimally invasive ankle reconstruction [56], and arthroscopic thermal-assisted capsular shift procedure [57].

The main procedures remain, however: Brostrom and its variations first described by Brostrom in 1965 [58] and 1966 [44], and modified and popularized by Gould in 1980 [45] and 1987 [59], and the Chrisman-Snook procedure first described in 1969 [60]. This is a modification of the Elmslie procedure with a long-term follow-up study published in 1985 [50].

Brostrom-Gould procedure

This is usually considered in acute ruptures or in chronic ATFL or CFL deficiency, with pain where preservation of the peroneal tendon and muscle group is required, for example in dancers, gymnasts, and athletes. Other authors have described the technique.

Results have been described in a number of publications. Gould and colleagues [45] were able to assess 50 of the 165 patients in their series, all scoring 8 to 10 in the scoring system they devised, with the score improving with time. Javors and colleagues [61] had 13 good or excellent results in 15 patients. Hamilton and colleagues [62] performed 28 operations, mainly in athletes and ballet dancers, and had 26 excellent results, one good and one fair result, at an average of 64.3 months follow-up. Messer and colleagues [63] reported good or excellent results in 16 of 22 patients using suture anchors. In the only randomized controlled trial available, Karlsson and colleagues [64] compared their own technique with Brostrom's. In 60 patients with a minimum follow-up of 2 years, 90% were good or excellent in their group, with 83% good or excellent in the Brostrom group.

Chrisman-Snook procedure

This is considered indicated in chronic ATFL or CFL deficiency particularly in obese patients, heavy sportsman, for example, rugby players, and in those with hindfoot deformity, which may be corrected. Concerns have been raised that ankle flexibility is not restored [65], and that subtalar motion is ablated without achieving ankle stability [66]. Other authors have used the technique.

Savastano and colleagues [67] described good or excellent results in an "athletic population." Snook and colleagues [50] published results in 48 cases with a 10-year mean follow-up. There were 45 good or excellent results. In a randomized controlled trial comparing Chrisman-Snook with the Brostrom-Gould [68] in 40 patients, the results were good or excellent in more than 80% in each group, with a slightly better outcome and fewer complications with the Brostrom-Gould technique.

McBride and colleagues

This technique is described as an alternative to other peroneus brevis tenodeses. It is an attempt at anatomic restoration, and may be combined with a translational os calcis (TOC) or alternative hindfoot osteotomy in patients without significant tilt of the talus or secondary osteoarthritis. The effect on the subtalar joint appears clinically minimal, but biomechanical tests are being evaluated. The technique is usually performed through a lateral incision in the interneural plane with a separate miniextended lateral approach for the TOC osteotomy if required (Fig. 6). The TOC osteotomy is performed with lateral displacement, which is usually achieved with relative ease. Two Kirschner wires have been used to maintain the position, but a single screw or double screw would be an alternative. The peroneus brevis tendon is harvested, and the anterior portion is used as in the Chrisman-Snook procedure but most recently as a free graft. Two drill holes are made in the distal fibula, the first from posterior to inferior to the tip of the fibula (Fig. 7), and the second more proximally running from posterior to anterior, that is, to the anterior distal edge of the fibula (Fig. 8). The CFL is reconstructed by using the initial inferior hole, and the tendon is passed from posterior to anterior through the superior drill hole to reconstruct the ATFL. This may be anchored using heavy absorbable sutures to the adjacent soft tissue and residual ATFL or by using suture anchors to the talus (Fig. 9). In the first few patients the tendon was left attached distally, but more recently it was detached and secured to the lateral wall of the os calcis using suture anchors. The peroneal retinaculum is then closed.

Results

In a preliminary study, 45 procedures were performed in 43 patients (23 males and 20 females) of a mixed athletic ability. We studied pain, stability, and whether or not the patient would have the procedure again. The American Orthopaedic Foot and Ankle Society (AOFAS) hindfoot scores were evaluated. The average follow-up was 6.5 years. The procedure resulted in adequate pain relief, stability, and return to sporting activity in 93%, all

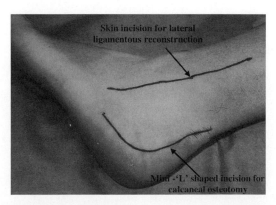

Fig. 6. Skin incisions for lateral ligamentous reconstruction and calcaneal osteotomy.

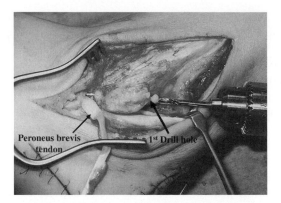

Fig. 7. Direction of the first drill hole in the fibula.

of this group stating, "they would have the operation again." The AOFAS hindfoot scores improved to an average of 89. Complications included two temporary sural nerve dysfunctions and a superficial wound infection, with all the TOC osteotomies healing uneventfully. There were two failures; each patient had hypermobility with a high body mass index (BMI). They were revised using fine synthetic grafts with effective results.

Postoperative care

Irrespective of the type of procedure, there has been a significant trend over the last 15 years away from cast immobilization to functional bracing and early rehabilitation [69]. A reasonable postoperative regime may include 2 weeks in a plaster backshell or Aircast boot until suture removal, followed by a further 6 weeks in the Aircast boot with early passive and active ankle

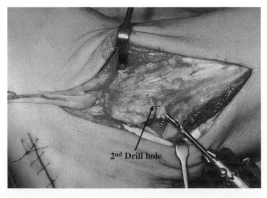

Fig. 8. Direction of the second drill hole in the fibula.

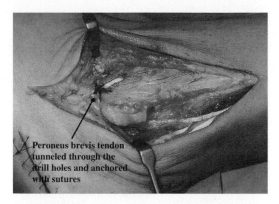

Peroneus brevis tendon tunneled through the drill holes and anchored with sutures

Fig. 9. Lateral ligamentous reconstruction with peroneus brevis tendon.

and subtalar mobilisation. Return to sporting activity will depend on patient preference, but is likely to be 3 to 6 months, depending on the sport and professional or amateur status.

Management of chronic ligamentous dysfunction with a varus tibiotalar joint

This is a demanding clinical condition, which remains difficult to treat.

Prevention

Ideally, and theoretically, one should be able to prevent this entity from developing. However, it remains controversial how this may be achieved. The evidence suggests a lower threshold for surgical repair in Grade III acute ligament ruptures [2]. Also, there are premorbid anatomic and functional factors, which may be identified. Adequate reconstruction in selected patients leads to a better outcome. However, our patients do not read the literature, and most present in early middle age with the established combination of ligamentous insufficiency, varus tilt of the talus in the mortise with or without secondary osteoarthritis to a greater or lesser degree, and frequently, subtalar osteoarthritis.

Conservative management

A not insignificant number of patients will prefer conservative management if they consider that the risks outweigh the benefits. They may also be hesitant about surgery when advised about the protracted postoperative course and recovery time. This group may include some elderly patients, and those with significant comorbidity, such as diabetes mellitus, peripheral vascular disease, certain neurologic disorders, cardiovascular, and respiratory disease.

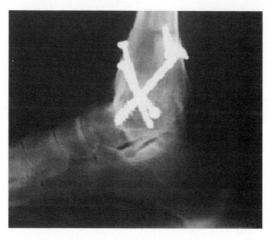

Fig. 10. Ankle arthrodesis.

Conservative management for those who wish to avoid surgery may include attention to footwear and the use of orthotics or traditionally callipers or braces. Pain relief using analgesia or anti-inflammatory medication may be appropriate, as may local anesthetic and corticosteroid injections, or a below-knee cast for the more acute episodes. Modification of lifestyle, in particular, sporting activity, may be sufficient for others.

Surgical management

In those patients who prefer surgery for adequate pain relief and stability the traditional management has been an ankle arthrodesis (Fig. 10) with

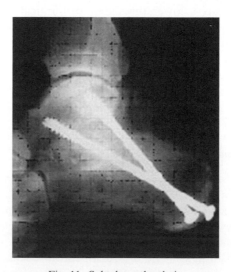

Fig. 11. Subtalar arthrodesis.

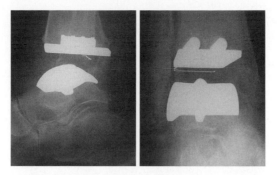

Fig. 12. Ankle replacement.

a hindfoot osteotomy if the subtalar joint is unaffected. In most patients, the subtalar joint is stiff because of secondary involvement, and a transcalcaneal–talar–tibial fusion using an intramedullary nail has been recommended. The situation is more complicated in patients who wish ankle mobility for work or leisure-related reasons. A hindfoot osteotomy with or without a corrective subtalar arthrodesis (Fig. 11) and ankle arthroscopy with debridement may appease some patients at least for a limited time, but correction of the deformity may be difficult. If this deformity can be corrected to within 20° of malalignment, ankle replacement (Fig. 12) has been advocated [70]. The most exciting developments recently, however, have been in relation to the use of external fixators. An Ilizarov frame with a footplate has been proposed by some, but is not as versatile as the Taylor Spatial Frame (Figs. 13 and 14). Once adequate correction of the hindfoot deformity has been achieved, arthroscopic debridement may be considered. Ankle replacement for patients with intractable osteoarthritic pain is an option.

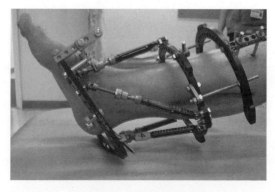

Fig. 13. Taylor spatial frame.

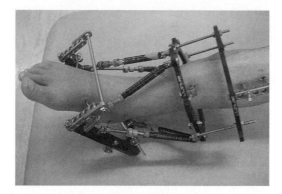

Fig. 14. Taylor spatial frame.

Summary

Many techniques have been described in acute and chronic lateral ligament insufficiency in the ankle. At present, the Brostrom-Gould and Chrisman-Snook procedures and their variations remain the "gold standard." Recent assessment of important etiologic factors has shed some light on the relationship between the original injury or injuries and the subsequent development of the varus tibiotalar joint with or without secondary osteoarthritis. The development of the Taylor Spatial Frame may well revolutionize its management. In the meantime, further consideration should be given to well-designed and evaluated randomized controlled trials, improved understanding of the biomechanics, and function of the ligaments, for example, proprioceptive function and their healing. Newer and less invasive arthroscopic and percutaneous techniques are being developed.

References

[1] Schuberth JM, Collman DR, Rush SM, et al. Deltoid ligament integrity in lateral malleolar fractures: a comparative analysis of arthroscopic and radiographic assessments. J Foot Ankle Surg 2004;43(1):20–9.
[2] Pijnenburg AC, Van Dijk CN, Bossuyt PM, et al. Treatment of ruptures of the lateral ankle ligaments: a meta-analysis. J Bone Joint Surg Am 2000;82(6):761–73.
[3] Harrington KD. Degenerative arthritis of the ankle secondary to long-standing lateral ligament instability. J Bone Joint Surg Am 1979;61(3):354–61.
[4] Keefe DT, Haddad SL. Subtalar instability. Etiology, diagnosis and management. Foot Ankle Clin 2002;7(3):577–609.
[5] Sugimoto K, Samoto N, Takakura Y, et al. Varus tilt of the tibial plafond as a factor in chronic ligament instability of the ankle. Foot Ankle Int 1997;18(7):402–5.
[6] Fortin PT, Guettler J, Manoli A 2nd. Idiopathic cavovarus and lateral ankle instability: recognition and treatment implications relating to ankle arthritis. Foot Ankle Int 2002;23(11):1031–7.
[7] Van Bergeyk AB, Younger A, Carson B. CT analysis of hindfoot alignment in chronic lateral ankle instability. Foot Ankle Int 2002;23(1):37–42.

[8] Valderrabano V, Hintermann B, Horisberger M, et al. Ligamentous posttraumatic ankle osteoarthritis. Am J Sports Med 2006;34(4):612–20.

[9] Scranton PE Jr, McDermott JE, Rogers JV. The relationship between chronic ankle instability and variations in mortise anatomy and impingement spurs. Foot Ankle Int 2000; 21(8):657–64.

[10] Berkowitz MJ, Kim DH. Fibular position in relation to lateral ankle instability. Foot Ankle Int 2004;25(5):318–21.

[11] Lofvenberg R, Karrholm J, Selvik G. Fibular mobility in chronic lateral instability of the ankle. Foot Ankle 1990;11(1):22–9.

[12] Keeman JN. Commentaar Enkelspecial. Reuma Trauma 1990;1:34–5.

[13] Van Dijk CN. On diagnostic strategies in patients with severe ankle sprain. Thesis, Universiteit Van Amsterdam, Amsterdam; 1994.

[14] Zeegers AVCM. Het supinatie van de enkel. Thesis, Universiteit Van Utrecht, Utrecht; 1995.

[15] Peters JW, Trevino SG, Renstrom PA. Chronic lateral ankle instability. Foot Ankle 1991; 12(3):182–91.

[16] Karlsson J, Lansinger O. Lateral instability of the ankle joint. Clin Orthop Relat Res 1992; 276:253–61.

[17] Colville MR, Marder RA, Boyle JJ, et al. Strain measurement in lateral ankle ligaments. Am J Sports Med 1990;18(2):196–200.

[18] Larsen E, Lund PM. Peroneal muscle function in chronically unstable ankles. A prospective preoperative and postoperative electromyographic study. Clin Orthop Relat Res 1991;272: 219–26.

[19] Hartsell HD, Spaulding SJ. Eccentric/concentric ratios at selected velocities for the invertor and evertor muscles of the chronically unstable ankle. Br J Sports Med 1999;33(4): 255–8.

[20] Hiller CE, Refshauge KM, Beard DJ. Sensorimotor control is impaired in dancers with functional ankle instability. Am J Sports Med 2004;32(1):216–23.

[21] McVey ED, Palmieri RM, Docherty CL, et al. Arthrogenic muscle inhibition in the leg muscles of subjects exhibiting functional ankle instability. Foot Ankle Int 2005;26(12): 1055–61.

[22] Michelson JD, Hutchins C. Mechanoreceptors in human ankle ligaments. J Bone Joint Surg Br 1995;77(2):219–24.

[23] Lofvenberg R, Karrholm J, Sundelin G. Proprioceptive reaction in the healthy and chronically unstable ankle joint. Sportverletz Sportschaden 1996;10(4):79–83.

[24] Hintermann B. Biomechanics of the unstable ankle joint and clinical implications. Med Sci Sports Exerc 1999;31(7 Suppl):S459–69.

[25] Becker H, Rosenbaum D, Claes L, et al. Measurement of plantar pressure distribution during gait for diagnosis of functional lateral ankle instability. Clin Biomech (Bristol, Avon) 1997;12(3):S19.

[26] Nysaka M, Shabat S, Simkin A, et al. Dynamic force distribution during level walking under the feet of patients with chronic ankle instability. Br J Sports Med 2003;37:495–7.

[27] Liu W, Siegler S, Techner L. Quantitative measurement of ankle passive flexibility using an arthrometer on sprained ankles. Clin Biomech (Bristol, Avon) 2001;16(3):237–44.

[28] Hubbard TJ, Kaminski TW, Vander Griend RA, et al. Quantitative assessment of mechanical laxity in the functionally unstable ankle. Med Sci Sports Exerc 2004;36(5):760–6.

[29] Monaghan K, Delahunt E, Caulfield B. Ankle function during gait in patients with chronic ankle instability compared to controls. Clin Biomech (Bristol, Avon) 2006;21(2):168–74.

[30] Myerson MS. Surgery of disorders of the foot and ankle. London: Martin Dunitz Ltd.; 1996.

[31] Larsen E, Angermann P. Association of ankle instability and foot deformity. Acta Orthop Scand 1990;61(2):136–9.

[32] Boardman DL, Liu SH. Contribution of the anterolateral joint capsule to the mechanical stability of the ankle. Clin Orthop Relat Res 1997;341:224–32.

[33] Hasegawa A, Kimura M, Tomizawa S, et al. Separated ossicles of the lateral malleoulus. Clin Orthop Relat Res 1996;330:157–65.

[34] Busconi BD, Pappas AM. Chronic, painful ankle instability in skeletally immature athletes. Ununited osteochondral fractures of the distal fibula. Am J Sports Med 1996;24(5):647–51.

[35] Kanbe K, Hasegawa A, Nakajima Y, et al. The relationship of the anterior drawer sign to the shape of the tibial plafond in chronic lateral instability of the ankle. Foot Ankle Int 2002; 23(2):118–22.

[36] McKinley TO, Rudert MJ, Koos DC, et al. Incongruity versus instability in the etiology of posttraumatic arthritis. Clin Orthop Relat Res 2004;423:44–51.

[37] Frost SC, Amendola A. Is stress radiography necessary in the diagnosis of acute or chronic ankle instability? Clin J Sport Med 1999;9(1):40–5.

[38] Helagson JW, Chandnani VP. MR arthrography of the ankle. Radiol Clin North Am 1998; 36(4):729–38.

[39] Kirby AB, Beall DP, Murphy MP, et al. Magnetic resonance imaging findings of chronic lateral ankle instability. Curr Probl Diagn Radiol 2005;34(5):196–203.

[40] Trnka HJ, Ivanic G, Trattnig S. Arthrography of the foot and ankle. Ankle and subtalar joint. Foot Ankle Clin 2000;5(1):49–62.

[41] Komenda GA, Ferkel RD. Arthroscopic findings associated with the unstable ankle. Foot Ankle Int 1999;20(11):708–13.

[42] Hintermann B, Boss A, Schafer D. Arthroscopic findings in patients with chronic ankle instability. Am J Sports Med 2002;30(3):402–9.

[43] Okuda R, Kinoshita M, Morikawa J, et al. Arthroscopic findings in chronic lateral ankle instability: do focal chondral lesions influence the results of ligament reconstruction. Am J Sports Med 2005;33(1):35–42.

[44] Brostrom L. Sprained ankles. VI. Surgical treatment of "chronic" ligament ruptures. Acta Chir Scand 1966;132(5):551–65.

[45] Gould N, Seligson D, Gassman J. Early and late repair of lateral ligament of the ankle. Foot Ankle 1980;1(2):84–9.

[46] Rudert M, Wulker N, Wirth CJ. Reconstruction of the lateral ligaments of the ankle using a regional periosteal flap. J Bone Joint Surg Br 1997;79(3):446–51.

[47] Watson-Jones R. Fractures and joint injuries. 3rd edition. Baltimore (MD): Williams and Wilkins; 1946.

[48] Elmslie RC. Recurrent subluxation of the ankle joint. Ann Surg 1934;100:364.

[49] Evans DL. Recurrent instability of the ankle: a method of surgical treatment. Proc R Soc Med 1953;46:343.

[50] Snook GA, Chrisman OD, Wilson TC. Long-term results of the Chrisman-Snook operation for reconstruction of the lateral ligaments of the ankle. J Bone Joint Surg Am 1985;67(1):1–7.

[51] Sugimoto K, Takakura Y, Kumai T, et al. Reconstruction of the lateral ankle ligaments with bone-patellar tendon graft in patients with chronic ankle instability: a preliminary report. Am J Sports Med 2002;30(3):340–6.

[52] Takahashi T, Nakahira M, Kaho K, et al. Anatomical reconstruction of chronic lateral ligament injury of the ankle using pedicle tendon of the extensor digitorum longus. Arch Orthop Trauma Surg 2003;123(4):175–9.

[53] Westlin NE, Vogler HW, Albertsson MP, et al. Treatment of lateral ankle instability with transfer of the extensor digitorum brevis muscle. J Foot Ankle Surg 2003;42(4):183–92.

[54] Jeys LM, Harris NJ. Ankle stabilisation with hamstring autograft: a new technique using interference screws. Foot Ankle Int 2003;24(9):677–9.

[55] Coughlin MJ, Schenck RC, Grebing BR, et al. Comprehensive reconstruction of the lateral ankle for chronic instability using a free gracilis graft. Foot Ankle Int 2004;25(4):231–41.

[56] Wassermann LR, Saltzmann CL, Amendola A. Minimally invasive ankle reconstruction: current scope and indications. Orthop Clin North Am 2004;35(2):247–53.

[57] Hyer CF, Vancourt R. Arthroscopic repair of lateral ankle instability by using the thermal-assisted capsular shift procedure: a review of 4 cases. J Foot Ankle Surg 2004;43(2):104–9.

[58] Brostrom L. Sprained ankles. 3. Clinical observations in recent ligament ruptures. Acta Chir Scand 1965;130(6):560–9.

[59] Gould N. Repair of lateral ligament of the ankle. Foot Ankle 1987;8(1):55–8.

[60] Chrisman OD, Snook GA. Reconstruction of lateral ligament tears of the ankle. An experimental study and clinical evaluation of seven patients treated by a new modification of the Elmslie procedure. J Bone Joint Surg Am 1969;51(5):904–12.

[61] Javors JR, Violet JT. Correction of chronic lateral ligament instability of the ankle by use of the Brostrom procedure. Clin Orthop Relat Res 1985;198:201–7.

[62] Hamilton WG, Thompson FM, Snow SW. The modified Brostrom procedure for lateral ankle instability. Foot Ankle 1993;14(3):180.

[63] Messer TM, Cummins CA, Ahn J, et al. Outcome of the modified Brostrom procedure for chronic lateral ankle instability using suture anchors. Foot Ankle Int 2000;21(12):996–1003.

[64] Karlsson J, Eriksson BI, Bergsten T, et al. Comparison of two anatomic reconstructions for chronic lateral instability of the ankle joint. Am J Sports Med 1997;25(1):48–53.

[65] Tohyama H, Beynnon BD, Pope MH, et al. Laxity and flexibility of the ankle following reconstruction with the Chrisman-Snook procedure. J Orthop Res 1997;15(5):707–11.

[66] Rosenbaum D, Becker HP, Wilke HJ, et al. Tenodeses destroy the kinematic coupling of the ankle joint complex. A three-dimensional in vitro analysis of joint movement. J Bone Joint Surg Br 1998;80(1):11–2.

[67] Savastano AA, Lowe EB Jr. Ankle sprains: surgical treatment for recurrent sprains. Report of 10 patients treated with the Chrisman-Snook modification of the Elmslie procedure. Am J Sports Med 1980;8(3):208–11.

[68] Hennrikus WL, Mapes RC, Lyons PM, et al. Outcomes of the Chrisman-Snook and modified-brostrom procedures for chronic lateral ankle instability. A prospective, randomised comparison. Am J Sports Med 1996;24(4):400–4.

[69] Karlsson J, Lundin O, Lind K, et al. Early mobilisation versus immobilisation after ankle ligament stabilisation. Scand J Med Sci Sports 1999;9(5):299–303.

[70] Wood P, Deakin S. Total ankle replacement. The results in 200 ankles. J Bone Joint Surg Br 2003;85(3):334–41.

ELSEVIER
SAUNDERS

Foot Ankle Clin N Am
11 (2006) 625–637

FOOT AND
ANKLE CLINICS

Deltoid Ligament Injuries:
Diagnosis and Management

Beat Hintermann, MD*, Markus Knupp, MD,
Geert I. Pagenstert, MD

*Department of Orthopaedic Surgery, Orthopaedic Clinic, University of Basel, Kantonsspital
Liestal, CH-4410 Liestal, Switzerland*

The medial ligaments of the ankle are injured more often than generally believed [1,2]. These injuries can occur while running downstairs, landing on uneven surface, and dancing with the body simultaneously rotating in the opposite direction, thus sustaining a pronation (eversion) trauma (eg, an outward rotation of the foot during simultaneous inward rotation of the tibia). Excessive lateral rotation may injure the tibiofibular and interosseous ligaments at the syndesmosis. The anterior fibers of the deltoid ligament may also be involved in extreme rotation injuries. In practice, however, patients often report having sustained one or more ankle sprains, but they are unable to clearly indicate the mechanism of injury.

Complete deltoid ligament tears are occasionally seen in association with lateral malleolar fractures [3] or bimalleolar fractures [4].

Chronic deltoid ligament insufficiency can be seen in several conditions, including posterior tibial tendon disorder, trauma- and sports-related deltoid disruptions, and valgus talar tilting in patients who have a history of triple arthrodesis or total ankle arthroplasty.

One concern may be whether posterior tibial dysfunction and medial ankle instability are distinct conditions. Although possible, it is not clear yet whether—or to what extent—medial instability of the ankle may cause secondary posterior tibial tendon dysfunction, because the tendon may become elongated and/or may rupture [5].

This article focuses on the anatomy and function of the medial ligaments of the ankle and establishes a rationale for the diagnosis and treatment of incompetent deltoid ligament.

* Corresponding author.
E-mail address: b.hintermann@bluewin.ch (B. Hintermann).

1083-7515/06/$ - see front matter © 2006 Elsevier Inc. All rights reserved.
doi:10.1016/j.fcl.2006.08.001

Anatomy of the deltoid ligament

Wide variations have been noted in the anatomic description of the medial ligamentous complex of the ankle. This is a multibanded complex. Nevertheless, it is considered as having superficial and deep components [6]. The superficial ligaments cross two joints, namely the ankle and the subtalar joints. The deep ligaments cross only the ankle joint. However, this differentiation is not always absolutely clear [6]. During anatomic preparation of 40 cadavers, 6 different component bands were identified: 4 superficial (tibiospring, tibionavicular, superficial posterior tibiotalar, and tibiocalcaneal ligaments), of which only the tibiospring and tibionavicular ligaments were constant, and 2 deep bands (deep posterior tibiotalar and deep anterior tibiotalar ligaments), of which only the deep posterior tibiotalar ligament was constant. Boss and Hintermann [7] differentiated 3 superficial and more anterior bands (tibionavicular, tibiospring, and tibiocalcaneal ligaments) and 3 deep bands (anterior, intermediate, and posterior tibiotalar ligaments).

Because the tibioligamentous portion of the superficial deltoid has a broad insertion on the "spring ligament," this ligament complex may interplay with the deltoid ligament to stabilize the medial ankle joint, and thus functionally not be separated from it (Fig. 1).

Function of deltoid ligament

The deltoid ligament is a strong restraint-limiting talar abduction [8]. With all lateral structures removed, the intact deltoid ligament allows only 2 mm of separation between the talus and medial malleolus. When the deep deltoid ligament is released, the talus can be separated from the medial malleolus by 3.7 mm. Grath [9] confirmed these findings in a similar experiment. Rasmussen and colleagues [10,11] investigated the

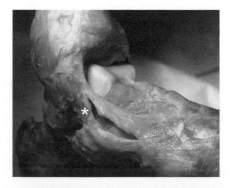

Fig. 1. Anterior aspect of the superficial bundles of the deltoid ligament. The tibiospring ligament (*asterisk*) has a broad insertion to the deltoid ligament.

function of various parts of the deltoid ligament. The superficial layers of the deltoid ligament specifically limit talar abduction or negative talar tilt. The talocalcaneal ligament specifically limits talar pronation, while the deep layers of the deltoid ligament rupture in external rotation without the superficial portion being involved. The deltoid ligament is the primary restraint against pronation of the talus, with the superficial and deep components equally effective [12]. Nigg and colleagues [13] stated that the deltoid ligament appears to be sensitive to plantar flexion, external rotation, and pronation.

Clinical presentation of incompetence of the deltoid ligament

Acute injuries to the deltoid ligament must be suspected after an eversion and/or pronation injury. Typically, the foot is firm on the ground when an eversion force causes a valgus stress to the ankle, or an internal rotation force causes a pronation stress to the hindfoot. Acute injuries to the deltoid ligament can also occur in association with lateral ankle fracture. Chronic injuries to the deltoid ligament typically cause medial ankle instability. This must be suspected if the patient feels the ankle "give way," especially medially, when walking on even ground, downhill, or downstairs, or if the patient experiences pain at the anteromedial or lateral aspect of the ankle, especially on dorsiflexion of the foot [2].

Clinical findings

Acute injuries may present with tenderness and hematoma along the deltoid ligament. A key finding in chronic injuries of the deltoid ligament is pain in the medial gutter, typically provoked by palpation of the anterior border of medial malleolus [1,2]. With the patient bearing weight, excessive valgus of the hindfoot and pronation of the affected foot indicates laxity of the medial aspect of the ankle [1,2,5]. Typically, the excessive valgus of the hindfoot and pronation of the foot (Fig. 2A,C) disappears when the patient is asked to to activate the posterior tibial muscle (Fig. 2B,D). Analogously, the excessive valgus of the hindfoot and pronation of the foot (Fig. 2E) disappears when the patient is asked to go on tiptoes (Fig. 2F). Because there is no flattening of the medial longitudinal arch, hindfoot valgus and forefoot abduction are not corrected by performing the single heel rise test. In this way, posterior tibial dysfunction can easily be excluded.

A reliable clinical test is performed with the patient seated on an examination couch with the feet hanging free [2]. The heel of the affected ankle is gently grasped with one hand, and the tibia with the other hand. First, a varus and then a valgus tilt stress are applied to the heel, and the results compared are with the contralateral side. Second, an anterior drawer stress is performed, and the result is compared with the contralateral side.

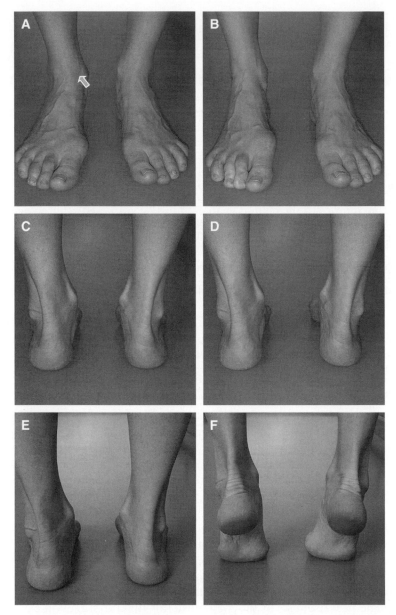

Fig. 2. This 39-year-old female sustained a pronation trauma to her right hindfoot while running on stairs 14 months before presenting to our clinic. Typically, she experienced pain in the medial gutter. (*A*) The arrow shows the medial gutter. (*B*) Frontal view of the patient when activating the tibialis posterior muscle. (*C*) Back view of normal stance. (*D*) Back view with the patient activating the tibialis posterior muscle. (*E*) Back view of normal stance. (*F*) Back view of the patient on tiptoes.

Imaging

Plain radiographs are used to exclude a fracture or other bony patholo-gies. In chronic conditions, weight-bearing radiographs to assess the extent of deformity if present. This is particularly true for a valgus deformity of the hindfoot as a result of a severe incompetence of medial ligaments of the ankle (Fig. 3).

Stress radiographs are helpful to gain indirect evidence of lesions of the deltoid ligament in the management of acute ankle fractures [4]. This is not the case in chronic conditions [2].

Arthrography has been used to detect acute tears of the deltoid ligament [14]. This method has mostly a historical interest at present.

If a talo-calcaneal coalition or a bony lesion involving the articular surfaces are suspected, CT is indicated. Although MRI may reveal injuries to the deltoid ligament, particularly acutely (Fig. 4A), we do not advocate the use of MRI on a regular basis.

Therefore, the criteria for diagnosing medial instability of the ankle are a feeling of "giving way," pain on the medial gutter, and a valgus and pro-nation deformity of the foot that can typically be corrected by the action of the tibialis posterior muscle.

Arthroscopic assessment

Ankle arthroscopy is helpful to confirm clinically suspected instability of the medial (Figs. 4B and 5) and lateral aspects of the ankle, and to detect additional pathologies such as cartilage lesions [2,15]. The ankle joint is graded as: (1) stable when there is some translocation of the talus, but not

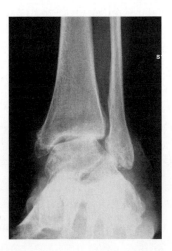

Fig. 3. This 54-year-old patient sustained a pronation trauma 2 years before presenting to our clinic. The weight-bearing anteroposterior view shows a market valgus tilt of the talus within the ankle mortise.

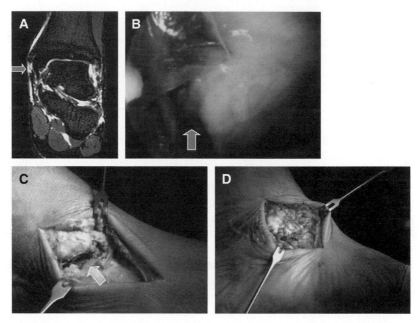

Fig. 4. An acute tear of the anterior superficial bundles of the deltoid ligament, including the tibionavicular, tibiospring, and tibiocalcaneal ligaments in a 26-year-old soccer player after pronation trauma. (*A*) MRI reveals the avulsion from the medial malleolus (*arrow*), whereas the deep tibiotalar ligaments are intact. (*B*) Arthroscopy reveals the detachment of these ligaments (*arrow*) from the anterior aspect of the medial malleolus. (*C*) At surgery, an extended horizontal tear of the anterior three bundles (superficial layer; *arrow*) of the deltoid ligament is evident. (*D*) The continuity of the ligament is restored after reconstruction of the ligament.

enough to open the tibiotalar joint by more than 2 mm, as measured by the 2 mm hook, and not enough to introduce the 5 mm arthroscope into the tibiotalar space; (2) moderately unstable when the talus subluxes out of the ankle mortise, allowing to introduce the 5 mm arthroscope into the tibiotalar space, but not enough to open the tibiotalar joint by more than 5 mm; and (3) severely unstable when the talus moves easily out of the ankle mortise, typically allowing for free access into the posterior aspect of the ankle joint without significant traction being applied on the heel [15].

Interestingly, 75% of patients who have chronic medial instability of the ankle show an associated avulsion of the anterior talofibular ligament that results in a complex rotational instability of the talus within the ankle mortise [2].

Surgical exploration of the medial ligaments of the ankle

Surgical exploration of the medial ligaments of the ankle should be performed in patients with symptomatic ankle instability in whom medial ankle instability has been suspected clinically and confirmed arthroscopically. If

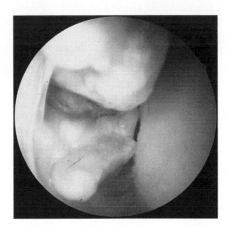

Fig. 5. Arthroscopic image of the medial ankle showing complete avulsion of the deltoid ligament.

additional instability of the lateral ankle ligament is suspected, the lateral ankle ligaments should also be explored.

On the medial side, a gently curved incision 4 to 8 cm long is made, starting 1 to 2 cm cranially of the tip of the medial malleolus toward the medial aspect of the navicular. After dissection of the fascia, the anterior aspect of the deltoid ligament is exposed. A longitudinal incision of the tendon sheath allows exploration of the tibialis posterior tendon and identification of the spring ligament. The tibionavicular ligament and the tibiospring ligament can then be explored.

The lateral ankle ligaments are exposed through a skin incision 5 to 8 cm long. The sinus tarsi and the subtalar joint are exposed and opened first. The dissection continues in a proximal direction while preserving the remaining and often scarred ligaments. The state of the stumps of the anterior talofibular ligament, calcaneofibular ligament, and lateral talocalcaneal ligament can then be assessed.

Classification of medial instability of the ankle

Medial ankle instability can result from an acute injury to the deltoid ligament and can include a wide injury pattern from partial to complete tearing of the ligament structures. Chronic medial ankle instability can, however, result from various conditions: an ankle sprain that has left residual instability of the talus within the mortise (eg, where the repetitive stress has worn out the superficial anterior bundles of the deltoid ligament), an insufficiency of the tibialis posterior muscle following tendon dysfunction (eg, where an increased valgus and pronation movement of the hindfoot is initiated while loading the foot), or a chronic overload in fixed valgus and flatfoot deformity (eg, where the acting valgus forces overcome the tensile properties of the deep tibiocalcaneal bundles of the deltoid ligament). We divide [1] injuries to the anterior bundles of the deltoid ligament into three lesion types: type I, in which there is a proximal tear or avulsion of the deltoid ligament; type II, in which there is an intermediate tear of the deltoid ligament; and type III, in which there is a distal tear or avulsion of the deltoid and spring ligaments.

Surgical techniques for medial ankle ligaments

Complete acute rupture

Complete acute rupture often occurs in the proximal portion of the deltoid ligament. Reinsertion to the medial malleolus is achieved by suturing directly to the bone (Fig. 4D). A bony anchor can also be used.

Chronic rupture of superficial deltoid ligament (type I lesion)

The anterior border of the medial malleolus is exposed by a short longitudinal incision between the tibionavicular and the tibiospring ligaments, where usually a small fibrous septum without adherent connective fibers between the two ligaments is present. After roughening of the medial aspect of the medial malleolus, an anchor is placed 6 mm above the tip of the malleolus, and used for fixation of the tibionavicular and tibiospring ligaments to the medial malleolus. In this way, both of these ligaments are retensioned. Additional heavy absorbable sutures are used to reinforce the repair.

Chronic rupture of superficial deltoid ligament (type II lesion)

The scarred insufficient ligament is divided into two flaps. The deep flap remains reattached distally, whereas the superficial flap remains reattached to the medial malleolus [1]. One anchor is placed 6 mm above the tip of the malleolus, and one anchor is placed at the superior edge of the navicular tuberosity. The two anchors serve to refixate the deep flap to the medial malleolus and the superficial flap to the navicular tuberosity, thereby producing a strong, well-tensioned reconstruction.

Additional heavy absorbable sutures are used to further stabilize the reconstructed tibionavicular and tibiospring ligaments.

Chronic rupture of superficial deltoid ligament (type III lesion)

If necessary, the tear is debrided [1]. Two nonabsorbable sutures are then placed in the spring ligament, and, if the tibionavicular ligament is completely detached from its insertion, an anchor is placed at the superior edge of the navicular tuberosity. After having tightened the sutures, additional heavy absorbable sutures are used to further stabilize the reconstructed tibionavicular and spring ligaments.

Chronic rupture of deep deltoid ligament

This condition most often includes an extended tear of the superficial anterior bundles of the deltoid ligament; therefore, any reconstructive procedure should address the entire deltoid ligament. The tibialis posterior tendon can be used as a graft for augmentation of the reconstructed deltoid ligament passing it through a drill hole from the tip of medial malleolus to the medial aspect of the distal tibia (Fig. 6). However, this technique does not sufficiently reinforce the deep tibiotalar ligaments (Hintermann, unpublished data). Recently, the use of a bone–tendon–bone graft has been proposed to reconstruct the deltoid ligament [16]. In this in vitro study, two limbs were created on the distal grat: one was fixed to the medial aspect of talus, the other to the sustentaculum tali. The proximal end of the graft was fixed either to the distal tibia, medial malleolus, or lateral tibia. Less than 2.0° of angulation was found while applying valgus stress of 5 daN for all fixation methods. However, the authors advised against fixation the proximal limb in the medial malleolus.

Additional procedures

The posterior tibial tendon is meticulously inspected during surgery, especially in a type II and type III lesion of the anterior deltoid ligament. If the tendon is degenerated, it is debrided. If the tendon is elongated, shortening of the tendon is considered. If there is an accessory bone (os tibiale externum), reattachment of the bone with the tendon insertion is considered. The tibialis posterior tendon can additionally be tightened if the bone is reattached more distally to the navicular bone [17]. A tendon transfer might be considered if more extensive tendon damage or frank tears are present.

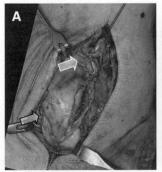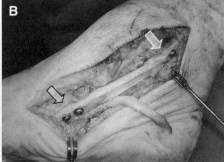

Fig. 6. Deltoid ligament reconstruction. (*A*) The tendon of the posterior tibialis is inserted in a drill hole into the medial malleolus (*black arrow*) and fixed to the periosteum of the distal tibia (*white arrow*). (*B*) Deltoid ligament reconstruction with a free bone–tendon–bone graft fixed distally to the medial cuneiform (*black arrow*) and proximally to the posterior aspect of the distal tibia (*white arrow*).

Reconstruction of the lateral ligamentous complex of the ankle is considered in the case of an additional lateral instability of the ankle. If the condition of the anterior talofibular ligament and calcaneofibular ligament allows an adequate primary repair, these ligaments are reconstructed by shortening and reinsertion. When no substantial ligamentous material is present, augmentation with a free plantaris tendon graft is performed.

A calcaneal lengthening osteotomy is considered if there is pre-existing valgus and pronation deformity of the foot (eg, when a valgus and pronation deformity is also present on the contralateral, asymptomatic foot), and/or in patients with severe attenuation or defect of the tibionavicular, tibiospring or spring ligaments. A calcaneal osteotomy is performed along and parallel to the posterior facet of the subtalar joint, from lateral to medial, preserving the medial cortex intact [18,19]. As the osteotomy is widened, the pronation deformity of the foot disappears. A tricortical graft from the iliac crest is fashioned to the length required, and placed into the osteotomy site.

A triple arthrodesis is considered when the medial ankle instability is so pronounced that a valgus tilt of talus within the mortise is seen on anteroposterior standard views of the ankle with the foot weight bearing (Fig. 3). Attention has to be paid to fully correct the entire deformity (eg, valgus malalignment of the heel and peritalar dislocation of the talus).

Postoperative management

The foot is protected in a plaster cast for 6 weeks, and allowed for full weight bearing as soon as pain allows. Rehabilitation starts afterward, with passive and active mobilization of the ankle joint, muscle training, and protection by a removable boot when walking. A walker or stabilizing shoe may be recommended for 4 to 6 weeks after plaster removal, depending on the muscle balance of the hindfoot. Afterward, we recommend its use for walks on uneven ground, high-risk sports activities, and professional work outdoors. If a triple arthrodesis is performed, initial plaster immobilization of 8 weeks is recommended.

The authors' experience

In an arthroscopic assessment of 288 acute ankle fractures, the deltoid ligament was injured more frequently than expected, particularly in Weber type B fractures [3]. Such injuries may be a source of persisting pain or pronation deformity when not appropriately treated. Although some authors believe that reconstruction of a ruptured deltoid ligament is not necessary [20], we advise careful reconstruction of the medial ligaments of the ankle if restoration of full mechanical stability is not proven after internal fixation of the fracture. This would be the case, for example, when repositioning of talus within the ankle mortise cannot be achieved because of interposition of the disrupted ligament between the medial malleolus and the talus.

Complete acute rupture of the deltoid ligament can also be seen in athletes after a valgus trauma, without injury to the lateral aspect of the ankle, though this is rare [14]. Because primary operative repair (Fig. 4) was found to produce satisfying results, we continue to consider surgical reconstruction in these acute injuries.

Chronic incompetence of the anterior superficial deltoid ligament causes chronic disabling pain and subjective instability [2]. In a prospective series of 52 patients, pain in the medial gutter was found in all ankles (100%), pain along the posterior tibial tendon was found in 14 ankles (27%), and pain along the anterior border of the lateral malleolus was found in 13 ankles (25%). A proximal rupture (type I lesion) of the deltoid ligament was noted in 37 patients (71%), an intermediate rupture (type II lesion) was noted in 5 patients (10%), and a distal rupture (type III lesion) was noted in 10 patients (19%). The tendon of the posterior tibialis was elongated in 6 patients (12%) and exhibited degeneration in 5 patients (10%), with no patients showing attenuation or rupture. Repair of the deltoid ligament was performed in all 52 patients, repair of the spring ligament was performed in 13 patients (24%), repair of the lateral ligaments was performed in 40 patients (77%), and an additional calcaneal lengthening osteotomy was performed in 14 patients (27%). At a mean follow-up of 4.4 years (range: 2.0–6.6), the AOFAS hindfoot score [21] had improved from 42.9 points preoperatively to 91.6 points. The clinical result was considered good to excellent in 46 cases (90%), fair in 4 cases (8%), and poor in 1 case (2%). Based on these favorable results, we have continued with this protocol. However, we consider additional calcaneal osteotomy (eg, medial sliding osteotomy to correct heel valgus, or lateral column lengthening osteotomy to correct pronation deformity of the hindfoot) more frequently, particularly in patients who have pre-existing deformities.

The greatest challenge is chronic incompetence of the deep deltoid ligament, which results in valgus tilt of the talus while bearing weight on the foot. Most attempts of isolated ligament reconstruction have failed, despite of the use of tendon augmentation; therefore, the preferred treatment is triple fusion to obtain a stable and well-aligned hindfoot. An alternative approach is tibiocalcaneal arthrodesis.

Summary

Recent work has shed more light on deltoid ligament injuries. The mechanism of injury can vary from an acute eversion stress to a repetitive rotational movement of the unstable talus within the ankle morise. Of 52 patients, 22 patients (42%) indicated they had sustained primarily a supination trauma, but thereafter they sustained other sprains; whereas 18 patients

(35%) reported having sustained an eversion trauma, and the other 12 patients (23%) reported having sustained one or multiple ankle sprains, but they were not able to clearly indicate the injury mechanism [2]. While increased pronation of the affected foot was found in 26 patients (50%), a similar deformity was also found in the contralateral unaffected foot in 11 patients (19%). Therefore, an acute ankle sprain may involve the deltoid ligament, particularly in eversion trauma. Recurrent ankle sprains after an initial inversion trauma can lead to incompetence of the anterior deltoid ligament which, in turn, increases sagittal plane movement of the medial talus within the ankle mortise. Furthermore, a pronation deformity of the foot may cause the deltoid ligament to wear out, resulting in incompetence.

The clinical manifestation of chronic medial ankle instability after injury to the deltoid ligament is a persisting valgus and/or pronation deformity of the hindfoot. Such ligamentous incompetence can be suspected based on the patient's feeling of having the ankle "give way," especially medially, when walking on even ground, downhill, or downstairs; pain at the anteromedial aspect of the ankle; and, occasionally, pain on the lateral aspect of the ankle, especially on dorsiflexion of the foot. The hallmark of the disorder is pain over the medial gutter of the ankle and a valgus and pronation deformity of the foot. The deformity can typically be actively corrected by the action of the tibialis posterior muscle. Arthroscopy is helpful for the diagnosis of medial instability. MRI, on the other hand, may help to detect associated cartilage lesions.

Surgical management of acute tears of deltoid ligament is recommended if the status of the remaining ligament structures against valgus stress cannot be proven. In chronic injuries of the superficial deltoid ligament with symptomatic medial instability of the ankle, surgical reconstruction should include all involved ligaments at the medial, and, if necessary, lateral aspect of the ankle. In the case of progressive foot deformity or bilateral long-standing valgus and pronation deformity of the foot, an additional calcaneal-lengthening osteotomy should be considered. If the chronic injury involves the deep deltoid ligament, isolated ligament reconstruction may be critical but could potentially fail if anatomic alignment of the hindfoot has not been achieved by way of osteotomy and/or triple fusion. In the case of severe valgus deformity, tibiocalcaneal arthrodesis may be considered.

References

[1] Hintermann B. Medial ankle instability. Foot Ankle Clin 2003;8:723–38.
[2] Hintermann B, Valderrabano V, Boss AP, et al. Medial ankle instability—an exploratory, prospective study of 52 cases. Am J Sports Med 2004;32:183–90.
[3] Hintermann B, Regazzoni P, Lampert C, et al. Arthroscopic findings in acute fractures of the ankle. J Bone Joint Surg Br 2000;82:345–51.
[4] Tornetta P III. Competence of the deltoid ligament in bimalleolar ankle fractures after medial malleolar fixation. J Bone Joint Surg Am 2000;82:843–8.

[5] Nelson DR, Younger A. Acute posttraumatic planovalgus foot deformity involving hind-foot ligamentous pathology. Foot Ankle Clin 2003;8:521–37.

[6] Milner CE, Soames RW. The medial collateral ligaments of the human ankle joint: anatomical variations. Foot Ankle Int 1998;19:289–92.

[7] Boss AP, Hintermann B. Anatomical study of the medial ankle ligament complex. Foot Ankle Int 2002;23:547–53.

[8] Close JR. Some applications of the functional anatomy of the ankle joint. J Bone Joint Surg 1956;38A:761–81.

[9] Grath G. Widening of the ankle mortise. A clinical and experimental study. Acta Orthop Scand 1960;263(Suppl):1–88.

[10] Rasmussen O. Stability of the ankle joint: analysis of the function and traumatology of the ankle ligaments. Acta Orthop Scand 1985;56(Suppl):1–75.

[11] Rasmussen O, Kroman-Andersen C, Boe S. Deltoid ligament: functional analysis of the medial collateral ligamentous apparatus of the ankle joint. Acta Orthop Scand 1983;54:36–44.

[12] Harper MC. Deltoid ligament: an anatomical evaluation of function. Foot Ankle 1987;8:19–22.

[13] Nigg BM, Skarvan G, Frank CB, et al. Elongation and forces of ankle ligaments in a physiological range of motion. Foot Ankle 1990;11:30–40.

[14] Jackson R, Wills RE, Jackson R. Rupture of deltoid ligament without involvement of the lateral ligament. Am J Sports Med 1988;16:541–3.

[15] Hintermann B, Boss A, Schäfer D. Arthroscopic findings in patients with chronic ankle instability. Am J Sports Med 2002;30:402–9.

[16] Buman EM, Khazen G, Haraguchi N, et al. Minimally invasive deltoid ligament reconstruction: a comparison of three techniques. Presented at the Proceedings of the 36th Annual Winter Meeting, Speciality Day AOFAS. Chicago, March 25, 2006.

[17] Knupp M, Hintermann B. Reconstruction in posttraumatic combined avulsion of an accessory navicular and the posterior tibial tendon. Techn Foot Ankle Surg 2005;4:113–8.

[18] Hintermann B, Valderrabano V. Lateral column lengthening by calcaneal osteotomy. Techn Foot Ankle Surg 2003;2:84–90.

[19] Hintermann B, Valderrabano V, Kundert HP. Lengthening of the lateral column and reconstruction of the medial soft tissue for treatment of acquired flatfoot deformity associated with insufficiency of the posterior tibial tendon. Foot Ankle Int 1999;20:622–9.

[20] Stromsoe K, Hoqevold HE, Skjeldal S, et al. The repair of a ruptured deltoid ligament is not necessary in ankle fractures. J Bone Joint Surg 1995;77:920–1.

[21] Kitaoka HB, Alexander IJ, Adelaar RS, et al. Clinical rating systems for the ankle-hindfoot, midfoot, hallux, and lesser toes. Foot Ankle Int 1994;15:349–53.

ELSEVIER
SAUNDERS

Foot Ankle Clin N Am
11 (2006) 639–657

FOOT AND
ANKLE CLINICS

Acute and Chronic Syndesmosis Injuries: Pathomechanisms, Diagnosis and Management

Norman Espinosa, MD*, Jonathan P. Smerek, MD, Mark S. Myerson, MD

Institute for Foot and Ankle Reconstruction, Mercy Medical Center, 301 St. Paul Street, Baltimore, MD 21202, USA

Since their first description by Quenu in 1912, the recognition and management of syndesmotic injuries have remained controversial [1]. Although a significant amount of research has focused on injuries of the lateral ligamentous complex, the literature about syndesmosis injuries has been limited. Syndesmosis injuries have been reported in conjunction with ankle sprains to ankle fractures, with an incidence between 1% and 18% [2–4]. Although isolated ligamentous syndesmosis sprains are rare, syndesmotic injuries frequently are mis- or undiagnosed, resulting in chronic ankle pain, disability, and eventually arthritic changes in the ankle joint. This is best reflected by the work of Vincelette and coworkers [5,6], who observed that late calcifications of the distal tibiofibular syndesmosis were present in 32% of professional football players, reflecting a prior undetected syndesmosis lesion, suggesting that the actual incidence may be higher than reported.

The spectrum of injuries to the syndesmosis ranges from a simple sprain to frank diastasis. Bonnin defined the term diastasis as loosening of the attachments between tibia and fibula at the distal tibiofibular joint, and clearly stated that this is not necessarily confined to wide separation of the bones [7]. Hence, a sprain of the syndesmosis may occur without a fracture as well as without diastasis.

Syndesmotic injuries, especially isolated, can be difficult to diagnose. Also, a longer recovery period for athletes must be expected when compared with any other type of ankle sprain [2,6,8–10]. In the past, internal fixation of almost every syndesmosis injury was recommended [11–14]. More

---

* Corresponding author.
E-mail address: noresp@gmx.net (N. Espinosa).

1083-7515/06/$ - see front matter © 2006 Elsevier Inc. All rights reserved.
doi:10.1016/j.fcl.2006.07.006

recently, greater knowledge about the anatomy and biomechanics of the distal tibiofibular joint have led to new management strategies in both acute and chronic injuries. Anatomic restoration of the distal tibiofibular syndesmosis is essential to provide adequate function of the ankle and to prevent degenerative joint disease.

The present review focuses on the anatomy, biomechanics, diagnosis, and management options in both acute and chronic syndesmotic injuries.

Anatomy and biomechanics

The distal tibiofibular joint is comprised of the tibia and fibula, which are connected by four major ligamentous structures. Anteriorly, the anterior inferior tibiofibular ligament (AITFL) originates from the Tillaux-Chaput tubercle on the tibia and runs obliquely at an approximate angulation to the tibial plafond of 45° to insert on the anterior aspect of the distal shaft of the fibula. Its width averages 20 mm, with a length of approximately 20 to 30 mm. The interosseous ligament (IOL) lies 0.5 to 2 cm above the joint line. The IOL is the shortest, but primary, attachment between the tibia and fibula. At its superior aspect, the IOL merges with the interosseous membrane (IOM), which provides only minimal additional reinforcement of the syndesmotic complex. On the posterior aspect of the syndesmosis lies the posterior inferior tibiofibular ligament (PITFL), divided into a superficial (SPITFL) and deep portion. The superficial portion originates from the posterior tibial surface at the posterolateral tubercle. It courses obliquely to insert on the distal and posterior aspect of the fibula. The average width of the SPITFL is 20 mm, with a length of approximately 30 mm and a thickness of 5 mm. The deep portion, often defined as the transverse tibiofibular ligament (TTFL), lies anterior and inferior to the SPITFL. It forms the most distal aspect of the tibiotalar articulation and functions as a labrum.

The ankle undergoes triplanar motion from plantarflexion to dorsiflexion [15–17]. Some triplanar motion also occurs in the distal tibiofibular joint. During these movements, the talus and the malleoli remain in contact, requiring perfect adaptation of the mortise. The superior part of the talus is wider anteriorly than posteriorly. In dorsiflexion, the anterior part of the talus engages maximally with both malleoli, leading to highest stability of the ankle joint. The reverse happens in plantarflexion. The talus rotates externally an average of 5° to 6° during both active and passive ankle dorsiflexion. There is horizontal plane motion averaging 10° of external rotation and 7° of internal rotation [18,19]. The fibula moves approximately 2.4 mm distally during the stance phase of gait. These studies demonstrate that there is additional load and movement around the ankle joint, which must be absorbed. A 1-mm lateral shift of the talus was enough to cause a 42% decrease of contact area at the tibiotalar joint, with consequent increase of the transmitted peak pressures under such circumstances [20,21].

The syndesmotic ligaments help to maintain ankle stability, and their integrity is of great importance for this purpose. Sectioning studies showed that the AITFL provided 35%, the TTFL 33%, the IOL 22%, and the SPITFL 9% of the overall stability of the ankle [22], and failure of two of these ligaments leads to significant mechanical laxity of the syndesmosis. A recent cadaver study showed that dissection of the AITFL led to an average increase of the diastasis of 2.3 mm [23]. When sectioning the distal 8 cm of the IOL, an additional increase of 2.2 mm was found. Finally, when the PITFL was completely cut, the total amount of diastasis averaged 7.3 mm. Although Rasmussen and colleagues [18] were not able to show a significant increase of either external or internal rotation at the ankle, Xenos and colleagues [23] found a 10.2° increase in external rotation when all ligaments were sectioned.

Mechanism of injury

The most widely accepted mechanism resulting in injury of the syndesmotic ligaments is external rotation and hyperdorsiflexion. This mechanism is most common in the sports of American football and skiing. However, no single study has been able to reproduce isolated syndesmotic injuries when applying an external rotation moment at the ankle joint. Other mechanisms, such as eversion, inversion, plantarflexion, pronation, and internal rotation, have been reported. It is thought that in the neutral position, increasing external rotation at the ankle leads to stretching of the AITFL, resulting in its rupture. These forces are transmitted through the talus, which rotates externally and pushes against the fibula. While the fibula is forced into a more posterior position, the AITFL is tensioned. With further external rotation, the AITFL ruptures. Subsequently, the IOL or PITFL are stressed. The result is rupture of IOL and PITFL, even fracture of the fibula. During hyperdorsiflexion, the talus is forced into the mortise, with increasing mediolateral tension within the distal tibiofibular joint. The AITFL is thus stressed and may rupture. This mechanism, which is thought to be found in running and jumping sports, is rare.

Clinical evaluation

As in all injuries, thorough history and clinical examination are mandatory. History should result in relevant information about the mechanism of injury and current complaints of the patient. It is important to know the interval between injury and clinical presentation. This interval can be classified as acute (<3 weeks), subacute (3 weeks to 3 months), or chronic (>3 months).

Inspection may reveal swelling and bruising of the anterolateral aspect of the ankle. Any deformity is noted. Palpation is necessary to evaluate swelling and crepitus, which may indicate a fracture. In patients with an isolated syndesmosis injury, well-localized pain can be found anterior to the syndesmosis of the ankle. The physician should palpate the whole length of the fibula and both malleoli to rule out an associated bony or ligamentous injury.

The "squeeze test" [2] is performed squeezing the fibula at the midcalf. Pain exerted by this test may indicate syndesmotic injury. Recent works show, however, that this test is not reliable enough to diagnose a syndesmosis injury. A far more reliable test is the external rotation test of the foot [6]. The patient is sitting in front of the physician with the hips and knees flexed at 90°. The foot is held in neutral position, and the foot is grasped. Gentle external rotation is applied, and pain is highly suspicious for a syndesmosis injury.

Imaging

Conventional radiography

Plain radiographs, consisting of weightbearing anteroposterior (AP), lateral, and mortise views of the ankle, are essential. Up to 50% of all syndesmosis injuries include a bony avulsion (Fig. 1). Additionally, full-length AP and lateral views of the lower leg must be obtained to assess possible proximal fibular fractures. Bony avulsions may be localized at the anterior or posterior aspect of the tibia. In chronic injuries, a synostosis or calcification of the syndesmosis can be observed (Fig. 2).

The more reliable method in the acute setting to evaluate syndesmosis injury rests on determining the relationship between the distal tibia and fibula. In a cadaver study, Harper and Keller [24] determined the reliability of several different measurements of the tibiofibular syndesmosis. They recommended the following criteria to be consistent with a normal tibiofibular

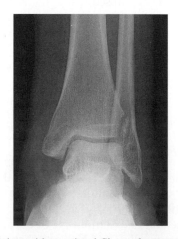

Fig. 1. Acute syndesmotic injury with associated Chaput fracture of the anterolateral aspect of the distal tibia.

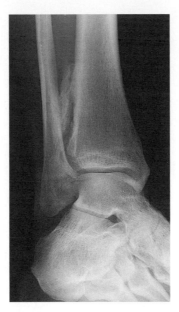

Fig. 2. Calcification within the syndesmosis, consistent with a clinical diagnosis of a chronic syndesmotic injury.

relationship: (1) a tibiofibular clear space of less than 6 mm on AP and mortise radiographs, (2) overlap of the tibia and fibula at the incisura fibularis tibiae of 6 mm or more or 42% or greater of the fibular width, and (3) overlap of the tibia and fibula greater than 1 mm on the mortise view. They concluded that the width of the tibiofibular clear space on both AP and mortise views appeared to be the most reliable variable for detecting early syndesmotic widening (Fig. 3). Six years later, Ostrum and colleagues [25] defined sex-specific absolute values and nonsex-specific ratios adjusting the values of Harper and Keller. Their new recommendations were as follows: (1) a tibiofibular clear space less than 5.2 mm in women and 6.5 mm in men, (2) a tibiofibular overlap of greater than 2.1 mm in females and 5.7 mm in males, (3) a ratio of tibiofibular overlap to fibular width greater than 24%, and (4) a ratio of tibiofibular clear space to fibular width of less than 44%. These values should help to determine the presence of posttraumatic disruption of the syndesmosis, and to assess mortise reduction postoperatively.

Stress radiography

Whereas frank diastasis is easy visible on radiographs, latent diastasis may easily go undetected. Although some authors recommended stress radiographs as a diagnostic adjunct, their usefulness remains questionable. Ogilvie-Harris and Reed [26] argued that stress radiography should be

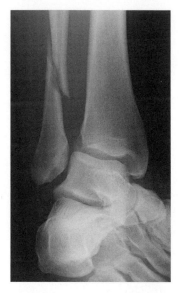

Fig. 3. Acute syndesmotic injury with no tibiofibular overlap on the mortise view.

used with caution, as they found 7 patients of 19 had a negative stress radio-graph, although arthroscopy provided evidence of syndesmotic injury. Xenos and colleagues [23] revealed that posterior displacement of the fibula on the lateral radiograph was more pronounced than the widening of the mortise on the AP view. However, definitive diagnosis of latent syndesmosis instability or injury may not be detected without additional diagnostic evaluation.

Bone scintigraphy

Bone scintigraphy of the ankle with technetium-99m pyrophosphate allows to evaluate occult syndesmosis injuries with 100% sensitivity, 71% specifity, and 93% accuracy in diagnosing a syndesmotic lesion in the absence of a fracture.

Computed tomography and magnetic resonance imaging

The advantage of computed tomography (CT) and magnetic resonance imaging (MRI) lies in the ability to produce three-dimensional images. The advantage of MRI over CT is the possibility of detection of concomitant injuries to the structures around and within the ankle [27,28]. Ebraheim and colleagues [29] used a cadaver model to demonstrate the superior impact of CT over conventional radiography. Routine radiographs were not able to detect 1 mm and 2 mm, diastases of the syndesmosis. All were detected by CT. Routine radiographs failed in 50% of all patients to identify 3-mm diastases. Takao and colleagues [28] compared the accuracy of standard AP radiography, mortise radiography, and MRI with arthroscopy of the ankle for the diagnosis of a tear of the syndesmosis in 52 patients. In comparison with arthroscopy, the sensitivity, specificity and accuracy were 44.1%, 100%, and 63.5% for standard AP radiography and 58.3%, 100%, and 71.2% for mortise radiography. In MRI, they were 100%, 93.1%, and 96.2% for a tear of the AITFL and 100%, 100%, and 100% for a tear of the PITFL. Standard AP and mortise radiographs did not always lead to the correct diagnosis [28]. Similar findings were also reported by Oae and colleagues [30].

Fixation techniques

Although screw fixation has been the standard management, there are still controversies regarding how distal tibiofibular fixation is performed. In a bio-mechanical study, there was less syndesmotic widening with screw placement 2.0 cm above the tibiotalar joint line when comparing with screw placement 3.5 cm proximal to the ankle joint line [31]. Kukreti and colleagues [32] retro-spectively evaluated the clinical and radiographic outcomes in two groups of patients: one had a syndesmotic screw placed through the syndesmosis itself, the other had a syndesmotic screw placed just above the syndesmosis. The two groups did not differ significantly in terms of clinical and radiographic out-comes. Beumer and associates assessed syndesmotic screw strength and fixa-tion capacity during cyclical testing in a cadaver model that simulated protected weight bearing [33]. They found no difference in fixation of the syndesmosis when stainless steel screws were compared with titanium screws through three or four cortices. They also concluded that the syndesmotic screw could not prevent excessive syndesmotic widening when loaded with a load comparable with body weight, and therefore, patients with a syndesmotic screw in situ should not bear weight.

The number of cortices engaged during fixation, as well as screw diame-ter, continues to elicit controversy. A recent prospective randomized study showed that fixation with two 3.5-mm tricortical screws provided better stability than fixation of the syndesmosis with one 4.5-mm quadricortical screw [34]. However, screw removal seems to be easier with quadricortical fixation. There was no biomechanical advantage of a single 4.5-mm screw when compared with a single 3.5-mm screw [35].This contrasts with the work by Hansen and colleagues [36], who demonstrated that a 4.5-mm quadricortical screw produced a higher yield load and peak load when compared with the 3.5-mm quadricortical syndesmotic screws. Based on these findings, they suggested that a larger diameter screw provides greater resistance to an applied shear stress at the distal syndesmosis.

Newer, absorbable fixation techniques are in use. Seitz and colleagues [37] described a new and flexible fixation technique using suture endobuttons. When compared with screw fixation, this technique is minimally invasive and provides semirigid and dynamic stabilization. The suture endobutton allows some external rotation and sagittal motion of the fibula. Recent works showed that there was a more consistent performance of the suture endobutton when compared with the standard AO-screw fixation technique, which demonstrated higher standard deviation values [38]. In a cadaveric study, they compared the suture-endobutton construct versus a single quadricortical 4.5-mm AO screw fixation. There were no significant differences in the mean rate of failure between the suture endobutton and AO screw fixation. The subsequent clinical trial of the same group demonstrated that the final clinical outcome in patients treated by the suture endobutton technique did not differ from those treated with screw fixation, and there was no need for implant removal [39]. Patients in whom the suture endobutton technique had been used had a faster rehabilitation. Thordarson and coworkers [40] presented the results of 17 patients who had fibular plate fixation with a 4.5-mm polylactic acid (PLA) bioabsorbable syndesmotic screw, and compared their results to 15 patients who had been treated by fibular plate fixation using a 4.5-mm stainless steel syndesmotic screw. In their series, all 32 patients had uncomplicated healing of their fibular fracture without loss of reduction. The group could not prove evidence of osteolysis nor sterile effusion in the patients who were treated with the PLA screw, and there were no wound complications in either group. Functional outcomes were similiar in terms of range of motion or subjective complaints. Again, as with the suture endobutton technique, no screw removal was necessary in the group with PLA. Similar results have been published by other authors [41–43], although some authors still report concerns in terms of screw breakage and removal.

Plate fixation has recently been described to enhance isolated syndesmosis fixation, and only a paucity of published reports exist. The addition of a plate increased compression forces across the syndesmosis in vitro, and led to higher rates of fusion in vivo [44]. However, this was shown in patients with total ankle arthroplasty. In their study, syndesmosis arthrodesis was the achieved goal. Most et al., (manuscript in preparation) in a cadaver study, investigated the effect of two-hole 3.5-mm one-third tubular plate fixation in simulated pronation–external rotation ankle fractures (high-fibula fracture Weber C), which involved disruption of the syndesmosis. The plate construct, including two 3.5-mm quadricortical screws, was compared with two 3.5-mm quadricortical fixation alone. Stability of the syndesmosis was tested via measurement of lateral displacement of the fibula, both during external rotation fatigue testing and in external rotation torque to failure. Failure torque was significantly higher in the screw-only group: the plate fixation was too rigid, and served as a stress riser, leading to earlier failure.

The current literature reports no definitive standard of fixation. As long as the syndesmosis can be reduced anatomically and be stable, any of the above described techniques could be considered: the only significant predictor of functional outcome is the amount and accuracy of syndesmotic reduction [45]. Therefore, personal preference and experience play an important role in choosing the fixation technique for the patient.

Management of acute syndesmosis injuries

Acute injuries to the syndesmotic complex can be divided in those involving only ligamentous structures and those associated with ankle fracture.

Acute and subacute isolated ligamentous injury

There is little published literature on the management of purely ligamentous syndesmotic injuries: these injuries are often mis- or undiagnosed, and subsequently are incorrectly rehabilitated.

Despite underdiagnosis, a conservative course of management is usually warranted. In a 1998 study, 96 cadets of the United States Military Academy underwent conservative management for ankle sprain injuries [46]. Sixteen cadets had an isolated syndesmotic injury. The final outcome for this group after 6 months was worse than those sustaining a lateral ligament sprain. In a 3-year prospective study, 60 consecutive collegiate athletes with "high" ankle symptoms over a 3-year period were all managed by a standard rehabilitation protocol, with an average time to return to full competitive activity of 13.4 days. The number of days missed from competition was statistically related to the length of interosseous tenderness, which was found to be an important premanagement criterium, and to positive results on the squeeze test. Six months after injury, 53 athletes were reevaluated. Patients rated their outcomes as good or excellent. Six of the patients experienced occasional ankle pain and stiffness, four patients reported recurrent ankle sprains, and one patient had heterotopic ossification formation. Taylor and coworkers [47] managed 44 football players conservatively: 23% of patients had chronic ankle pain, 36% ankle stiffness, and 18% had persistent swelling after an average follow up of 47 months. Patients with a longer recovery time showed ossification of the IOM. In regard to ankle function, the entire study population showed good to excellent results in 86%. Hopkinson and colleagues [2] also showed that patients with syndesmotic sprains had a siginificant longer recovery period.

Conservative management in patients with a sprained syndesmosis is functional, and consists of a walking boot or stirrup brace. In compliant patients, weight bearing as tolerated may be initiated immediately. Sometimes, though, pain predominates and crutches may be needed.

Patients with a latent diastasis, or with proven evidence of a reduced fibula in relation to the tibia, can be managed nonoperatively. Additionally, patients with frank diastasis demonstrated by a posteriorly subluxed or dislocated fibula, or superior subluxation or dislocation of the talus into the mortise, can be managed nonoperatively if longitudinal traction helps to reduce the fibula and the talus [48]. In these patients, immobilization in a nonweightbearing cast or walking boot for a period of 4 to 6 weeks is recommended. It is important to follow-up the reduction of fibula and talus in short-term intervals. After the initial 4 weeks, patients can start with partial weight bearing, and should reach full weight bearing after 8 weeks. Aggressive physical therapy is then started, with stretching, strengthening, range of motion and proprioceptive training to allow return to sport and daily activities.

Patients with latent diastasis and an irreducible fibula (as confirmed by CT or MRI) and those with frank diastasis (with possible plastic deformation of the fibula) may need open reduction and internal fixation with a screw [49,50]. No definitive literature exists clarifying the optimal management of these patients. In the series of Edwards and DeLee [50], six patients with acute syndesmosis injury underwent open reduction and internal fixation of the distal tibiofibular joint with a standard syndesmotic screw fixation with additional repair of the AITFL and the deltoid ligament. No recurrence was noted after screw removal. Fritschy demonstrated successful management of an isolated syndesmosis injury in 10 skiers [50a]. Three were treated surgically by open reduction and screw fixation. All patients returned to full activity and had no pain.

In patients with either acute or subacute syndesmosis injury, an attempt of direct repair of the torn AITFL in conjunction with screw fixation can be considered. Should a direct repair fail, reconstruction of the AITFL by means of autogenous (plantaris) or allograft tissue (hamstring) is a reasonable option.

Author's preferred management

The surgical approach relies on precise definition of the injured ligamentous complex. A longitudinal incision is made anteriorly over the distal tibiofibular joint space. All branches of the superficial peroneal nerve should be identified and protected. The tibiofibular space is directly visuatlise. The surgeon may find a torn AITFL, but should start with removal of the osteocartilagenous debris and interposed soft tissue. If there is an anterior avulsion fragment, it is important to determine whether it is large enough to allow stable fixation. If not, it is removed. If adequate reduction of the talus is not possible, then a deltoid ligament tear must be considered. In this instance, the soft-tissue interposition on the medial aspect of the ankle inhibits reduction of the talus. A separate medial incision may be necessary to free the medial clear space from soft tissue. However, in most patients there is no need for deltoid ligament repair. During reposition of the distal tibiofibular joint, repeated fluoroscopic checks are performed to ensure proper positioning before definitive fixation (Fig. 4A–C). We recommend using quadricortical 3.5-mm syndesmotic screws inserted parallel to the

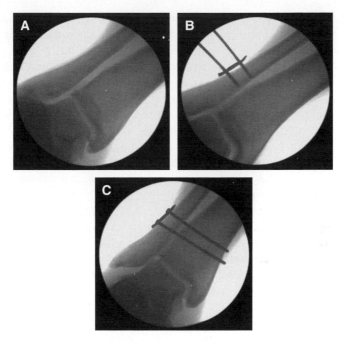

Fig. 4. (*A*) Fluoroscopic images demonstrating the approach to an isolated, acute syndesmotic disruption. (*B*) A two-hole 1/3-tubular plate is used to maximize compression between the fibula and tibia. The screws are inserted 2 cm above the plafond, parallel to the tibiotalar joint. (*C*) Final reduction is achieved while holding the ankle in maximal dorsiflexion.

ankle joint line from the posterolateral aspect of the fibula and directed at a 30° anterior angle into the tibia. The comparison with the normal side can help in determining anatomic reduction.

Postoperatively, a nonweightbearing cast is worn for 6 weeks. Screw removal is usually performed 3 months postoperatively, and aggressive rehabilitation is started. Physical therapy should focus on range of motion at the ankle, strengthening and proprioception. Patients should be counseled that recovery time might take up to 6 months.

Acute syndesmosis injury associated with ankle fracture

Ankle fractures, specifically Maisonneuve-, Weber-B, and Weber-C types, are often associated with rupture of the ligamentous complex of the syndesmosis. Leeds and Ehrlich [51] evaluated the late results after bimalleolar and trimalleolar ankle fractures in 34 patients after an average follow-up of 4 years. Of these patients, 21 patients had received open reduction and internal fixation of the medial malleolus only, and 13 internal fixation of both the medial and the lateral malleoli. There were significant correlations between (1) the adequacy of the reduction of the syndesmosis and late arthritis, (2) the accuracy of initial reduction of the syndesmosis and the late stability of the syndesmosis, (3) the late stability of the syndesmosis and the final outcome, and (4) the adequacy of the reduction of the lateral malleolus and that of the syndesmosis. Adequate reduction of the syndesmosis is mandatory to achieve a stable ankle following supination-external rotation and pronation-external rotation fractures of the ankle. The reduction of the syndesmosis will be unsatisfactory if the lateral malleolus is not well reduced.

Whereas the criteria for open reduction and internal fixation of ankle fractures is well defined, the need for syndesmotic fixation is less well understood. Often a syndesmotic screw is added, resulting in overmanagement. In 1994, Yamaguchi and colleagues [52] proposed a new protocol for the selected exclusion of trans-syndesmotic fixation in Weber C ankle fractures following a prospective study in 21 consecutive patients. They proposed that trans-syndesmotic fixation was not required if (1) rigid bimalleolar fracture fixation was achieved or (2) lateral without medial fixation was obtained if the fibular fracture was within 4.5 cm of the joint. They found that only 14% of the patients required trans-syndesmotic fixation. Ten patients did not receive trans-syndesmotic fixation. At 1- to 3-year follow-up intervals, no stress or static view widening of the mortise or syndesmosis was seen in any patient on conventional radiography. They concluded that, given their guidelines, trans-syndesmotic fixation was unnecessary in many patients. Its need could be determined preoperatively by assessing the integrity of the deltoid ligament and the level of the fibular fracture.

Multiple studies have attempted to address the need for syndesmotic fixation in patients with a deltoid rupture, as well as the level of fibula fracture. In a retrospective study performed, the factors affecting the outcome of Weber type-C ankle fractures in 43 patients were evaluated at 2 to 8 years follow-up [53]. Thirty-one patients underwent open reduction and internal fixation of the tibiofibular joint. Similar to Yamaguchi and colleagues, they assessed the use of a diastasis screw as appropriate or inappropriate based on the criteria by Boden and colleagues [54]. Interestingly, although the diastasis screw was used unnecessarily in 19 of the 31 patients in the study, this did not appear to affect the final functional result. The worse functional results were found in patients with dislocation of their ankles at time of injury, in patients with fractures of the medial malleolus, and in patients with deltoid ligament ruptures. Accurate reduction of the fibula and the syndesmosis led to better results. In contrast, a greater increase in the width of the syndesmosis was associated with a worse result. They suggested that an increase of more than 1.5 mm in syndesmosis width was unacceptable. If the deltoid ligament was torn, a diastasis screw should be used if the fibular fracture was more than 3.5 cm above the top of the syndesmosis. Additionally, in the presence of a fracture of the medial malleolus, which had been rigidly fixed, a diastasis screw would be required if the fibular fracture is located more than 1.5 cm above the syndesmosis. Similar findings were recently reported by Weening and colleagues. Of 425 ankle fractures, 51 required syndesmotic screw fixation [45]. At final follow-up, 16% of patients had unnecessary screw fixation, and improved ultimate outcome was only influenced when anatomic reduction of syndesmosis has been achieved. In 32 Weber C ankle fractures with fibular fractures above the distal tibiofibular syndesmosis [55] that underwent open reduction and internal fixation and were reevaluated at 25 months, syndesmotic screw fixation was added, which was removed after 9 weeks in 72% of fractures. In this series, 72% of patients had a good result, 13% had a fair, and 16% a poor result. Reduction and temporary fixation of the distal tibiofibular joint helped achieve fibular length to restore normal biomechanics of the ankle. As the five patients with poor results included three with syndesmotic diastasis with fibular nonunion, the authors advised not to remove the syndesmotic screw until there are signs of healing of the fibular fracture. Complex injuries were associated with higher rates of complications, and poor results in syndesmotic fixation could have been attributed to early removal of the syndesmotic screws. In a more recent study, the use of the level of fracture as a criterion for syndesmotic fixation has been questioned argued [56].

These data point to the fact that late syndesmotic instability and development of posttraumatic arthritis can be prevented with perfect and durable anatomic restoration of the mortise. If anatomic reduction cannot be established, the altered mechanics may enhance development of arthritis and impair final clinical outcome.

Screw removal

Early screw removal (6–8 weeks) postoperatively can be associated with failure of syndesmotic fixation [55,57]. Therefore, screw removal should be performed at the earliest 3 months postoperatively. This is not a strict recommendation, however. In very heavy patients, or in patients with poor compliance, the interval may be longer.

Chronic syndesmosis injuries

Syndesmotic instability can cause chronic, persistent ankle pain after a fracture or severe ankle sprain. Frequently, patients complain of a sensation of giving way and difficulty with walking on uneven ground [58]. Clinically, they present with stiffness, limited dorsiflexion, and persistent tenderness and swelling in the anterolateral aspect of the syndesmosis. Physical findings are unreliable, however, and the final diagnosis should be made in accordance with additional diagnostic imaging or arthroscopy [59]. Axial CT imaging provides great anatomic detail of the distal tibiofibular joint and is the most useful preoperative planning tool.

Management

Most published work on management strategy for chronic syndesmotic consists of case reports detailing a wide variety of approaches. Beals and Manoli [60] reported excellent results in a patient who presented 6 months from injury with persistent syndesmotic widening. He was treated with a medial arthrotomy for gutter debridement, resection of anterior tibiofibular scar tissue, and repair of the AITFL after reduction and fixation of the syndesmosis with a 6.5-mm screw with a washer. Similarly, Beumer and colleagues [61] described significant improvement in ankle scores in nine patients who underwent reconstruction with proximal and medial advancement of a bone block involving the tibial attachment of the slack AITFL. Harper [62] debrided the tibiofibular space and reduced the syndesmosis with one or two large four cortices syndesmotic screws. He did perform one arthrodesis due to painful popping. Five of six patients were completely satisfied at 1-year follow-up, with a period of nonweight bearing for 1 to 2 months and removal of hardware 12 to 28 weeks after surgery.

The presence of the syndesmotic adhesions have also been implicated as a source of chronic pain in syndesmotic injuries. Prisch and colleagues [63] treated 11 patients with chronic ankle pain 6 to 9 months after ankle fracture. All had dramtic pain relief with a 3-week return to prefracture functional capacity after aggressive arthroscopic excision of syndesmotic adhesions. He surmised that the nonphysiologic tissue limits motion and results in impingement of the hypertrophied tissue against the lateral talar dome in dorsiflexion.

Multiple procedures have been described to reconstuct the syndesmotic ligamentous complex. to avoid syndesmotic fusion, which may limit physiologic motion of the fibula, restrict talar motion, and result in ankle stiffness [64]. Grass and colleagues [65] described a technically demanding procedure of harvesting a portion of the peroneus longus and weaving it through bone tunnels to recreate the AITFL, IOL, and PITFL. At 16 months follow-up, all patients had relief of chronic swelling in the ankle and significant decrease in the tibiofibular clear space.

No studies have reported the outcome after isolated syndesmotic arthrodesis.The perception is that the procedure is limiting to patient, leading some surgeons to recommend it only as a salvage procedure. Pena and Coetzee [66] recommend arthrodesis after 6 months, and only if significant incongruency in seen on CT scan. If the injury is less than 6 month old, he recommends debridement of the syndesmosis and repeat screw fixation.Only after failure of screw fixation is arthrodesis attempted.

Author's preferred management

A chronic syndesmosis injury is defined as persistent syndesmotic widening 3 months after injury. At this time, the ruptured AITF, PITF, or IO ligaments have healed in an elongated position. Frequently, scar tissue is present in the medial gutter, which prevents the talus from seating anatomically in the mortise.

The approach to reconstruction follows a systematic approach from a medial to lateral direction. First, the medial gutter is debrided either arthroscopically or via a medial miniarthrotomy. If there is concomitant intraarticular pathology, such as an osteochondral defect, arthroscopic debridement is preferred. Otherwise, a miniarthrotomy makes removal of the dense scar tissue easier without the risk of articular cartilage damage

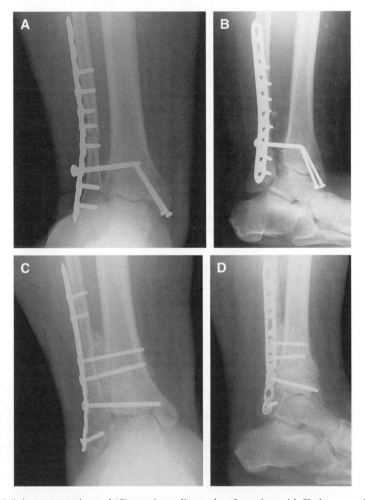

Fig. 5. (A) Anteroposterior and (B) mortise radiographs of a patient with fibular nonunion and chronic syndesmotic widening. The patient underwent a distal tibial realignment osteotomy, grafting, and compression of the fibular nonunion, and a syndesmosis fusion with allograft and iliac crest aspirate. Four-month follow-up (C) Anteroposterior and (D) mortise radiographs demonstrating a healed fibular nonunion and syndesmotic fusion. The patient had complete resolution of pain.

with arthroscopic instruments. The anterolateral distal syndesmotic space can be visualized arthroscopically, but, given the amount and density of the scar tissue, open debridement is preferred.

To approach the syndesmosis, an incision is made from the distal anterior aspect of the fibula extending 6 cm proximally along the anterior border. The superficial peroneal nerve is carefully retracted anteriorly at all times.The distal syndesmosis is aggressively debrided to remove all scar and soft tissue. The syndesmosis is subsequently sprung open with a lamina spreader. The lateral border of the tibia and the medial border of the fibula are decorticated with an AO chisel to promote bleeding cancellous bony surfaces. The interval is then copiously packed with crushed cancellous allograft and demineralized bone matrix. The syndesmosis is then clamped with ankle in maximal dorsiflexion. Finally, an anatomically contoured three- or four-hole 1.3 tubular plate is applied laterally to the fibula and fixed with two or three fully threaded 3.5-mm syndesmotic screws engaging four cortices (Fig. 5A–D). The postoperative protocol involves at least 6 to 8 weeks of nonweight bearing, depending on the time to fusion. Range of motion exercises are begun in 4 to 6 weeks.

Summary

Both acute and chronic syndesmotic injuries can lead to significant morbidity. The key to management of acute injuries is anatomic reduction of the fibula and the syndesmosis. A high index of suspicion for syndesmotic injuries will allow the surgeon to avoid the difficult reconstruction options for chronic diastasis.

References

[1] Quenu E. Du diastatsis de l'articulation tibio-peronier. Rev Chir 1912;45:416–38.
[2] Hopkinson WJ, St Pierre P, Ryan JB, et al. Syndesmosis sprains of the ankle. Foot Ankle 1990;10:325–30.
[3] Brostrom L. Sprained ankles. 3. Clinical observations in recent ligament ruptures. Acta Chir Scand 1965;130:560–9.
[4] Fallat L, Grimm DJ, Saracco JA. Sprained ankle syndrome: prevalence and analysis of 639 acute injuries. J Foot Ankle Surg 1998;37:280–5.
[5] Vertullo C. Unresolved lateral ankle pain. It's not always "just a sprain." Aust Fam Physician 2002;31:247–53.
[6] Boytim MJ, Fischer DA, Neumann L. Syndesmotic ankle sprains. Am J Sports Med 1991;19: 284–98.
[7] Bonnin J. Injuries to the ankle. London: W. Heinemann Medical Books Ltd; 1950.
[8] Wright RW, Barile RJ, Surprenant DA, et al. Ankle syndesmosis sprains in national hockey league players. Am J Sports Med 2004;32:1941–5.
[9] Wuest TK. Injuries to the distal lower extremity syndesmosis. J Am Acad Orthop Surg 1997; 5:172–81.
[10] Ward DW. Syndesmotic ankle sprain in a recreational hockey player. J Manipulative Physiol Ther 1994;17:385–94.

[11] Roberts RS. Surgical treatment of displaced ankle fractures. Clin Orthop Relat Res 1983;164–70.

[12] Pankovich AM. Fractures of the fibula at the distal tibiofibular syndesmosis. Clin Orthop Relat Res 1979;138–47.

[13] Pankovich AM. Maisonneuve fracture of the fibula. J Bone Joint Surg Am 1976;58:337–42.

[14] Weigert M, Luth A. Injury of the distal tibiofibular syndesmosis, its diagnosis and treatment. Z Orthop Ihre Grenzgeb 1967;103:199–210.

[15] Leardini A, O'Connor JJ, Catani F, et al. A geometric model of the human ankle joint. J Biomech 1999;32:585–91.

[16] Inman VT. The influence of the foot–ankle complex on the proximal skeletal structures. Artif Limbs 1969;13:59–65.

[17] Lapidus PW. Kinesiology and mechanical anatomy of the tarsal joints. Clin Orthop Relat Res 1963;30:20–36.

[18] Rasmussen O, Tovborg-Jensen I, Boe S. Distal tibiofibular ligaments. Analysis of function. Acta Orthop Scand 1982;53:681–6.

[19] Rasmussen O, Tovborg-Jensen I. Anterolateral rotational instability in the ankle joint. An experimental study of anterolateral rotational instability, talar tilt, and anterior drawer sign in relation to injuries to the lateral ligaments. Acta Orthop Scand 1981;52:99–102.

[20] Ramsey PL, Hamilton W. Changes in tibiotalar area of contact caused by lateral talar shift. J Bone Joint Surg Am 1976;58:356–7.

[21] Burns WC 2nd, Prakash K, Adelaar R, et al. Tibiotalar joint dynamics: indications for the syndesmotic screw—a cadaver study. Foot Ankle 1993;14:153–8.

[22] Ogilvie-Harris DJ, Reed SC, Hedman TP. Disruption of the ankle syndesmosis: biomechanical study of the ligamentous restraints. Arthroscopy 1994;10:558–60.

[23] Xenos JS, Hopkinson WJ, Mulligan ME, et al. The tibiofibular syndesmosis. Evaluation of the ligamentous structures, methods of fixation, and radiographic assessment. J Bone Joint Surg Am 1995;77:847–56.

[24] Harper MC, Keller TS. A radiographic evaluation of the tibiofibular syndesmosis. Foot Ankle 1989;10:156–60.

[25] Ostrum RF, De Meo P, Subramanian R. A critical analysis of the anterior–posterior radiographic anatomy of the ankle syndesmosis. Foot Ankle Int 1995;16:128–31.

[26] Ogilvie-Harris DJ, Reed SC. Disruption of the ankle syndesmosis: diagnosis and treatment by arthroscopic surgery. Arthroscopy 1994;10:561–8.

[27] Brown KW, Morrison WB, Schweitzer ME, et al. MRI findings associated with distal tibiofibular syndesmosis injury. AJR Am J Roentgenol 2004;182:131–6.

[28] Takao M, Ochi M, Oae K, et al. Diagnosis of a tear of the tibiofibular syndesmosis. The role of arthroscopy of the ankle. J Bone Joint Surg Br 2003;85:324–9.

[29] Ebraheim NA, Lu J, Yang H, et al. Radiographic and CT evaluation of tibiofibular syndesmotic diastasis: a cadaver study. Foot Ankle Int 1997;18:693–8.

[30] Oae K, Takao M, Naito K, et al. Injury of the tibiofibular syndesmosis: value of MR imaging for diagnosis. Radiology 2003;227:155–61.

[31] McBryde A, Chiasson B, Wilhelm A, et al. Syndesmotic screw placement: a biomechanical analysis. Foot Ankle Int 1997;18:262–6.

[32] Kukreti S, Faraj A, Miles JN. Does position of syndesmotic screw affect functional and radiological outcome in ankle fractures? Injury 2005;36:1121–4.

[33] Beumer A, Campo MM, Niesing R, et al. Screw fixation of the syndesmosis: a cadaver model comparing stainless steel and titanium screws and three and four cortical fixation. Injury 2005;36:60–4.

[34] Hoiness P, Stromsoe K. Tricortical versus quadricortical syndesmosis fixation in ankle fractures: a prospective, randomized study comparing two methods of syndesmosis fixation. J Orthop Trauma 2004;18:331–7.

[35] Thompson MC, Gesink DS. Biomechanical comparison of syndesmosis fixation with 3.5- and 4.5-millimeter stainless steel screws. Foot Ankle Int 2000;21:736–41.

[36] Hansen M, Le L, Wertheimer S, et al. Syndesmosis fixation: analysis of shear stress via axial load on 3.5-mm and 4.5-mm quadricortical syndesmotic screws. J Foot Ankle Surg 2006;45: 65–9.

[37] Seitz WH Jr, Bachner EJ, Abram LJ, et al. Repair of the tibiofibular syndesmosis with a flexible implant. J Orthop Trauma 1991;5:78–82.

[38] Thornes B, Walsh A, Hislop M, et al. Suture-endobutton fixation of ankle tibio-fibular diastasis: a cadaver study. Foot Ankle Int 2003;24:142–6.

[39] Thornes B, Shannon F, Guiney AM, et al. Suture-button syndesmosis fixation: accelerated rehabilitation and improved outcomes. Clin Orthop Relat Res 2005;207–12.

[40] Thordarson DB, Samuelson M, Shepherd LE, et al. Bioabsorbable versus stainless steel screw fixation of the syndesmosis in pronation-lateral rotation ankle fractures: a prospective randomized trial. Foot Ankle Int 2001;22:335–8.

[41] Hovis WD, Kaiser BW, Watson JT, et al. Treatment of syndesmotic disruptions of the ankle with bioabsorbable screw fixation. J Bone Joint Surg Am 2002;84-A:26–31.

[42] Sinisaari IP, Luthje PM, Mikkonen RH. Ruptured tibio-fibular syndesmosis: comparison study of metallic to bioabsorbable fixation. Foot Ankle Int 2002;23:744–8.

[43] Kaukonen JP, Lamberg T, Korkala O, et al. Fixation of syndesmotic ruptures in 38 patients with a malleolar fracture: a randomized study comparing a metallic and a bioabsorbable screw. J Orthop Trauma 2005;19:392–5.

[44] Jung HG, Nicholson JJ, Parks B, et al. Radiographic and biomechanical support for fibular plating of the agility total ankle. Clin Orthop Relat Res 2004;118–24.

[45] Weening B, Bhandari M. Predictors of functional outcome following transsyndesmotic screw fixation of ankle fractures. J Orthop Trauma 2005;19:102–8.

[46] Gerber JP, Williams GN, Scoville CR, et al. Persistent disability associated with ankle sprains: a prospective examination of an athletic population. Foot Ankle Int 1998;19: 653–60.

[47] Taylor DC, Englehardt DL, Bassett FH 3rd. Syndesmosis sprains of the ankle. The influence of heterotopic ossification. Am J Sports Med 1992;20:146–50.

[48] Clanton TO, Paul P. Syndesmosis injuries in athletes. Foot Ankle Clin 2002;7:529–49.

[49] Miller CD, Shelton WR, Barrett GR, et al. Deltoid and syndesmosis ligament injury of the ankle without fracture. Am J Sports Med 1995;23:746–50.

[50] Edwards GS Jr, DeLee JC. Ankle diastasis without fracture. Foot Ankle 1984;4:305–12.

[50a] Fritschy D. An unusual ankle injury in top skiers. Am J Sports Med 1989;17:282–5; discussion 285–6.

[51] Leeds HC, Ehrlich MG. Instability of the distal tibiofibular syndesmosis after bimalleolar and trimalleolar ankle fractures. J Bone Joint Surg Am 1984;66:490–503.

[52] Yamaguchi K, Martin CH, Boden SD, et al. Operative treatment of syndesmotic disruptions without use of a syndesmotic screw: a prospective clinical study. Foot Ankle Int 1994;15: 407–14.

[53] Chissell HR, Jones J. The influence of a diastasis screw on the outcome of Weber type-C ankle fractures. J Bone Joint Surg Br 1995;77:435–8.

[54] Boden SD, Labropoulos PA, McCowin P, et al. Mechanical considerations for the syndesmosis screw. A cadaver study. J Bone Joint Surg Am 1989;71:1548–55.

[55] Ebraheim NA, Mekhail AO, Gargasz SS. Ankle fractures involving the fibula proximal to the distal tibiofibular syndesmosis. Foot Ankle Int 1997;18:513–21.

[56] Ebraheim NA, Elgafy H, Padanilam T. Syndesmotic disruption in low fibular fractures associated with deltoid ligament injury. Clin Orthop Relat Res 2003;260–7.

[57] Harper MC. The deltoid ligament. An evaluation of need for surgical repair. Clin Orthop Relat Res 1988;156–68.

[58] Beumer A, Valstar ER, Barling EH, et al. Kinematics before and after reconstruction of the anterior syndesmosis of the ankle. Acta Orthop 2005;76(5):713–20.

[59] Beumer A, Swierstra BA, Mulder PG. Clinical diagnosis of syndesmotic ankle instability: evaluation of stress tests behind the curtains. Acta Orthop Scand 2002;73(6):667–9.

[60] Beals TC, Manoli A. Late syndesmotic reconstruction: a case report. Foot Ankle Int 1998; 19:485–7.

[61] Beumer A, Heijboer RP, Fontijne PJ, et al. Late reconstruction of the anterior distal tibiofibular syndesmosis. Acta Orthop Scand 2000;71(5):519–21.

[62] Harper MC. Delayed reduction and stabilization of the tibiofibular syndesmosis. Foot Ankle Int 2001;22:15–9.

[63] Pritsch M, Lokiec F, Sali M, et al. Adhesions of distal tibiofibular syndesmosis: a cause of chronic ankle pain after fracture. Clin Orthop Relat Res 1993;220–2.

[64] Ney R, Jend H-H, Schotag H. Tibiofibulare beweglichkeit und arthrose bei patienten mit postopertiven ossifikationen im syndesmosenbereich des oberen sprunggelenkes. Unfallchirurgie 1987;13(5):274–7.

[65] Grass R, Rammelt S, Biewener A, et al. Peroneus longus ligamentoplasty for chronic instability of the distal tibiofibular syndesmosis. Foot Ankle Int 2003;24:392–7.

[66] Pena FA, Coetzee JC. Ankle syndesmosis injuries. Foot Ankle Clin N Am 2006;11:35–50.

ELSEVIER
SAUNDERS

Foot Ankle Clin N Am
11 (2006) 659–662

FOOT AND
ANKLE CLINICS

Epidemiology of Sprains of the Lateral Ankle Ligament Complex

Nicholas Antonio Ferran, MBBS, MRCSEd,
Nicola Maffulli, MD, MS, PhD, FRCS (Orth)*

*Department of Trauma and Orthopaedic Surgery, Keele University School of Medicine,
Thornburrow Drive, Hartshill, Stoke on Trent ST4 7QB Staffs, United Kingdom*

Ankle sprain is one of the most common injuries encountered during sporting activity [1]. The vast majority of ankle sprains involve the lateral ligament complex, and are also referred to as inversion sprains [2]. Lateral ankle sprains are often undertreated, resulting in chronic pain, muscular weakness, and recurrent giving way [3]. Ankle sprains result in loss of playing time for professional athletes, and high costs of rehabilitation for their clubs. The burden placed on Accident and Emergency Departments can be remarkable.

The lateral ankle ligament complex consists of the anterior talofibular ligament (ATFL), the calcaneofibular ligament (CFL), and the posterior talofibular ligament (PTFL). The ATFL extends from the anterior–inferior border of the fibula to the neck of the talus. The CFL runs from the tip of the fibula to the lateral tubercle of the calcaneus. The PTFL extends from the digital fossa on the posterior border of the lateral malleolus to the lateral tubercle of the talus [4]. The ATFL is the weakest of the ligaments, and is involved in practically all lateral ankle sprains. The CFL is involved 50% to 75% of the time, and the PTFL in fewer than 10% [5]. The most common mechanism of injury is inversion, plantar flexion, and internal rotation. The relative shortness of the medial malleolus and the natural tendency for the ankle to go into inversion rather than eversion usually results in lateral ankle sprains [2].

Lateral ankle ligament injuries are graded from I to III [6], based on increasing ligamentous damage and morbidity. In a grade I sprain, the ATFL is stretched with some of the ligament fibers torn, but no frank ligamentous disruption is present. Clinically, the patient presents with mild swelling, little

* Corresponding author.
  E-mail address: n.maffulli@keele.ac.uk (N. Maffulli).

1083-7515/06/$ - see front matter © 2006 Elsevier Inc. All rights reserved.
doi:10.1016/j.fcl.2006.07.002

or no hematoma on the lateral aspect ankle, point tenderness on the ATFL, and no or mild restriction of active range of motion. Difficulty with full weight bearing is sometimes seen, and there is no laxity on examination.

A grade II sprain involves a moderate injury to the lateral ligamentous complex, frequently with a complete tear of the ATFL and an additional partial tear of the CFL. Examination shows restricted range of motion with localized swelling, echymosis, hemorrhage, and tenderness of the ante-rolateral aspect ankle. Abnormal laxity may be mild or may not be present. The patient experiences additional functional loss, with inability to toe rise or hop on the injured foot. A grade II injury may present with swelling and functional loss that makes it indistinguishable from a grade III injury in the acute setting.

A grade III injury implies complete disruption of both the ATFL and CFL, possibly with a capsular tear. An accompanying tear of the posterior talofibular ligament can be present. Examination often reveals diffuse swelling, echymosis on the lateral side of the ankle and heel, and tenderness over the anterolateral capsule, ATFL, and CFL. Moderate to severe laxity to an-terior drawer or inversion tests is usually present, but may not be elicited, de-pending on the amount of swelling and muscular spasm during examination.

When describing ankle sprains, the terms ankle ligament laxity, lateral ankle instability, and chronic ankle instability are often used interchange-ably. It is useful to define these terms to avoid confusion. Laxity is a physical sign objectively detected on examination, such as a positive anterior drawer or increased inversion. Lateral ankle instability is the presence of an unsta-ble ankle due to lateral ligamentous injury. The patient may describe this as the ankle giving way. Chronic ankle instability refers to repetitive episodes of instability resulting in recurrent ankle sprains [7].

In 1977, Garrick undertook a 2-year review of high school injuries; 14% of all injuries involved the ankle, with a rate of six injuries per 100 partici-pants. Of the ankle injuries, 85% were sprains (12% overall), and 80% of all ankle sprains involved the lateral ligaments of the ankle. Basketball, Amer-ican football, and women crosscountry running had the highest frequencies of ankle sprains [2]. In a study of first-time ankle sprains by Beynnon and colleagues [8], 4.8% of subjects suffered a sprain of the lateral ankle, that is, 0.85 injuries/1000 person days of exposure. This lower percentage com-pared with the Garrick study suggests a possible high frequency of recurrent sprains in the former study. The Beynnon study noted that there was no sig-nificant different in incidence rates between male and female athletes.

Ankle sprains often result in residual symptoms that can be troublesome, particularly to the professional athlete. In a survey of Hong Kong athletes with ankle sprains, 30.2% of injured athletes complained of residual pain. The second most common complaint was instability in 20.4% of athletes. The authors also found an increase in residual symptoms with increasing number of recurrent sprains. Athletes with multiple sprains complained of residual crepitus, weakness, instability, and stiffness. The athletes noted that residual symptoms affected their athletic performance to a greater degree with increasing number of recurrent sprains [3].

In a 2-year prospective study undertaken in the English Football Association, ankle sprains accounted for 11% of the injuries sustained. Seventy-seven percent of ankle sprains involved the lateral ligaments [9]. Ankle sprains accounted for 17% to 21% of all injuries sustained in a 1-year prospective study in the football leagues in Sweden [10]. In the English Football Association, one-third of ankle sprains were sustained during training, and two-thirds during matches. The impact of ankle sprains on clubs was significant: 12,138 days and 2033 matches were missed as a result. The reinjury rate for ankle sprains was 9%. Initial ankle sprains resulted in an average of 18 days and three matches missed, while reinjury resulted in an average of 19 days and four matches missed [9].

Although professional sports clubs and their medical teams may treat sprains sustained by their players, injuries in the general public tend to be managed by general practitioners and Accident and Emergency Departments. In a Danish prospective study of injuries presenting to a casualty ward, 4% of all injuries were due to foot and ankle sprains. An incidence of 7/1000 persons per year was estimated, for a total of 36,000 injuries in Denmark each year. Forty-five percent of injuries occurred during sport, 20% during play, and 16% during work. Males sustained their injuries more frequently during sport than females. Patients less than 25 years of age sustained more injuries on sports grounds, while patients over the age of 50 years sustained in-house accidents more frequently. Sixty-one percent of foot and ankle sprains were noted to involve the lateral ankle ligament complex [11]. In Accident and Emergency Departments in the West Midlands of the United Kingdom, an incidence rate of 60.9 ankle sprains per 10,000 persons was estimated. Fourteen percent of ankle sprains were classed as severe. When extrapolated to the UK population, this estimated 302,000 ankle sprains, of which 42,000 were severe [12].

Summary

Lateral ankle sprains account for 85% of all ankle sprains. This common injury is most frequently sustained during sporting activity. The ATFL is the weakest of the lateral ankle ligament complex, and is most frequently injured. Ankle sprains are often undertreated, resulting in chronic pain, muscular weakness, and instability. The consequence of this common injury for professional sports clubs is days lost in training and matches missed due to injury as well as the cost of rehabilitation. In the UK, an estimated 302,000 ankle sprains are seen each year in Accident and Emergency Departments.

References

[1] Beynnon BD, Murphy DF, Alosa DM. Predictive factors for lateral ankle sprains: a literature review. J Athl Train 2002;37(4):376–80.

[2] Garrick JG. The frequency of injury, mechanism of injury, and epidemiology of ankle sprains. Am J Sports Med 1977;5(6):241–2.

[3] Yeung MS, Chan KM, So CH, et al. An epidemiological survey on ankle sprain. Br J Sports Med 1994;28(2):112–6.

[4] Liu SH, Jason WJ. Lateral ankle sprains and instability problems. Clin Sports Med 1994; 13(4):793–809.

[5] Amendola A, Drosdewech D. Tendon and ligament disorders of the foot and ankle. In: Bulstrode C, et al, editors. Oxford textbook of orthopaedics and trauma. Vol. 2. New York: Oxford University Press; 2002. p. 1305–14.

[6] Chorley JN, Hergenroeder AC. Management of ankle sprains. Pediatr Ann 1997;26(1): 56–64.

[7] Hertel J. Functional anatomy, pathomechanics, and pathophysiology of lateral ankle instability. J Athl Train 2002;37(4):364–75.

[8] Beynnon BD, Vacek PM, Murphy D, et al. First-time inversion ankle ligament trauma: the effects of sex, level of competition, and sport on the incidence of injury. Am J Sports Med 2005;33(10):1485–91.

[9] Woods C, Hawkins R, Hulse M, et al. The Football Association Medical Research Programme: an audit of injuries in professional football: an analysis of ankle sprains. Br J Sports Med 2003;37(3):233–8.

[10] Ekstrand J, Tropp H. The incidence of ankle sprains in soccer. Foot Ankle 1990;11(1):41–4.

[11] Holmer P, Sondergaard L, Konradsen L, et al. Epidemiology of sprains in the lateral ankle and foot. Foot Ankle Int 1994;15(2):72–4.

[12] Bridgman SA, Clement D, Downing A, et al. Population based epidemiology of ankle sprains attending accident and emergency units in the West Midlands of England, and a survey of UK practice for severe ankle sprains. Emerg Med J 2003;20(6):508–10.

ELSEVIER
SAUNDERS

Foot Ankle Clin N Am
11 (2006) 663–683

FOOT AND
ANKLE CLINICS

Anterior and Posterior Ankle Impingement

C. Niek van Dijk, MD, PhD

*Academic Medical Center, University of Amsterdam, P.O. Box 22700,
1100 DD Amsterdam, The Netherlands*

Chronic anterior ankle pain is commonly caused by talotibial osteophytes at the anterior portion of the ankle joint. Morris [1], McMurray [2], and later Biedert [3], named this condition "athlete's" ankle or "footballer's" ankle, although it occurs in other sports, such as running, ballet dancing, high-jumping, and volleyball. The term "footballer's ankle" has been appropriately replaced by "anterior ankle impingement syndrome." Chronic posterior ankle pain is commonly caused by an os trigonum or other bony impediment, such as a hypertrophic posterior process of the talus.

The pain from impingement lesions is caused by synovial tissue being caught between the talus and the ankle mortise. Osteophytes or ossicles facilitate this process, because they limit the arc of motion. A differentiation has been made between soft tissue impingement and bony impingement lesions [3–5].

In general, osteophytes are the secondary manifestation of osteoarthritic changes [6,7]. However, repetitive minor trauma in the ankle, as seen in athletes, can induce spur formation [2], with radiographic characteristics similar to osteophytes.

In patients with anterior ankle impingement, recognizable pain on palpation is the most important clinical finding, while, for posterior impingement, recognizable pain on forced hyperplantarflexion is pathognomonic. When standard radiographs do not disclose the cause of an anterior impingement, special projections are used to disclose medially located bony spurs. When conservative management fails, surgery involves removal of bony or soft tissue impediments.

E-mail address: m.lammerts@amc.uva.nl

1083-7515/06/$ - see front matter © 2006 Elsevier Inc. All rights reserved.
doi:10.1016/j.fcl.2006.06.003

Etiology of anterior ankle impingement

Repeated capsuloligamentous traction by repetitive kicking with the foot in full plantarflexion may induce traction spurs formation [2]. This hypothesis is supported by the fact that these spurs are frequently found in athletes [2–4,8,9] who repetitively force their ankle in hyperplantarflexion actions, with repetitive traction to the anterior joint capsule [10]. It assumes, however, that the capsular attachment is located at the anterior cartilage rim at the location where spurs originate.

The anterior joint capsule attaches on the tibia at an average of 6 mm proximal to the joint level [11]. On the talar side, the capsule attaches likewise approximately 3 mm from the distal cartilage border. The distance of capsular attachment to the most frequent location of bony spurs is thus relatively large. Hence, the hypothesis of formation of talotibial traction spurs from recurrent traction to the joint capsule is not plausible. This is supported by observations at arthroscopy [12]. In patients with bony impingement, the location of tibial spurs is reported to be at the joint level, and always within the confines of the joint capsule [12,13]. On the talar side, the typical osteophytes are found proximal to the notch of the talar neck. Tibial and talar osteophytes can easily be detected at arthroscopy with the ankle in forced dorsiflexion. The capsule does not need to be detached to locate these osteophytes.

O'Donoghue [14] considered the osteophytes to be related to direct mechanical trauma associated with the impingement of the anterior articular border of the tibia and the talar neck during forced dorsiflexion of the ankle. Here, bone formation is considered to be a response of the skeletal system to intermittent stress and injury, as evidenced by Wolff's law of bone remodeling [15]. According to Hawkins [16] runners, dancers and high-jumpers are prime examples of athletes who may be predisposed to this type of sports-related repeated trauma. Even though this etiologic factor is widely cited [4,5,9,16], scientific evidence for either is scarce.

Along the distal tibia, the width of the nonweight-bearing cartilage rim extends up to 3 mm proximal to the joint line. It is this nonweight bearing anterior cartilage rim undergoes development of osteophytes [5,11]. Damage to this anterior cartilage rim occurs in the majority of supination trauma [17,18]. Depending on the amount of damage, chondral and bone cell stimuli will initiate a repair reaction may cartilage proliferation, scar tissue formation, and calcification. Additional damage by ankle sprains, due to recurrent instability or forced dorsiflexion movements, will further enhance this process [3]. Recent studies demonstrated that chronic ankle instability is indeed significantly correlated with osteophytic formation in the medial ankle compartment [18,19]. Another etiologic factor in the development of spurs is recurrent microtrauma. In soccer players, spur formation is related to recurrent ball impact, which can be regarded as repetitive microtrauma to the anteromedial aspect of the ankle [20]. Repetitive trauma to the anteromedial cartilage can probably be decreased by preventing recurrent ankle sprains.

In the anterior ankle impingement syndrome, the cause of pain is probably not the osteophyte itself, but the inflamed soft tissue caught between the traction spurs and the osteophytes [13]. The tibial and talar spurs typically do not overlap each other [21]. Histopathologic analysis of arthroscopic resected soft tissue reveals synovial changes and chronic inflammation [22]. In cadaver specimens, a triangular soft tissue synovial fold, subsynovial fat, and collagen tissue were found along the entire anterior tibiotalar joint line. This soft tissue component is squeezed between the anterior distal tibia and the talus during forced dorsiflexion. Recurrent trauma to this soft tissue may lead to hypertrophy of the synovial layer, subsynovial fibrotic tissue formation, and infiltration of inflammatory cells. Talar and tibial osteophytes decrease the anterior space, and compression of this soft tissue component is more likely to occur. It is therefore important to remove these osteophytes restoring the anterior space and reducing the chance that symptoms recur.

Posterior ankle impingement

Posterior ankle impingement can be caused by overuse or trauma. It is important to differentiate between these two, because posterior impingement from overuse has a better prognosis [23].

A posterior ankle impingement syndrome due to overuse is mainly found in ballet dancers and runners [7,24,25]. Running with forced plantarflexion, such as downhill running, can impose repetitive stresses on the posterior aspect of the ankle joint [25]. The forceful plantarflexion that occurs during the "en pointe" or the "demi-pointe" position produces compression at the posterior aspect of the ankle joint. Either of these situations can put extreme pressure on the anatomic structures normally present between the calcaneus and the posterior part of the distal tibia. Through exercise, the joint mobility and range of motion gradually increase, progressively reducing the distance between the calcaneus and the posterior portion of the distal tibia. Overall, if abnormal structures, such as a (slightly displaced) os trigonum, hypertrophic posterior talar process, a thickened posterior joint capsule, posttraumatic scar tissue, posttraumatic calcifications of the posterior joint capsule, a loose body in the posterior part of the ankle joint, or an osteophyte at the posterior distal tibia, are present, they may be compressed during hyperplantarflexion.

The presence of a prominent posterior talar process or os trigonum in itself is not sufficient to produce the syndrome. In 1995, we reported on a group of 19 retired dancers (mean age 59 years; range 50–66), and examined their ankle and subtalar joints [7]. The mean length of the ballet dancers' professional careers was 37 years. All the dancers had been dancing "en pointe" for an average of 45 hours a week. None of the ballet dancers had been free from injuries, but in none of them macrotrauma had occurred.

None of the dancers had experienced a posterior ankle impingement syndrome. In 18 of the 38 investigated ankle joints, a hypertrophic posterior talar process or os trigonum was present (Fig. 1). In most cases, the os trigonum was relatively large [7]. Therefore, the presence of an os trigonum or prominent talar process in itself does not seem to be relevant. An os trigonum must be combined with a traumatic event, such as a supination trauma, dancing on hard surfaces, or pushing beyond anatomic limits. The pain is caused by an abnormal movement between os trigonum and talus (Fig. 2), compression of thickened joint capsules or scar tissue between the os trigonum and tibia, or compression between os trigonum and calcaneus (known as "dancers' heel").

The posterior talar prominence becomes compressed between the tibia and the calcaneus during forced plantarflexion. In the presence of an os trigonum, this can lead to micromotion of the os trigonum, and pain (Fig. 3). A fracture can occur if the posterior talar process is prominent. Compression of the posterior joint capsule can lead to calcification. Combined supination and plantarflexion (leading to a lateral ankle ligament lesion) in some patients also leads to compression of posteromedially located joint structures. In these patients, the posttraumatic calcifications often are located posteromedially (Fig. 4).

Clinical features ankle impingement

Typically, patients with an anterior ankle impingement are relatively young athletes with recurrent inversion injuries of the ankle [26]. Patients

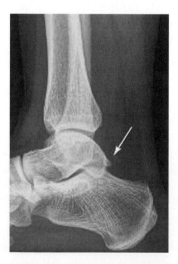

Fig. 1. Lateral X-ray of the left ankle of a 54-year-old female former professional ballet dancer having performed a professional career for over 40 years. No posterior ankle pain. *Arrow* indicates a prominent posterior talar process.

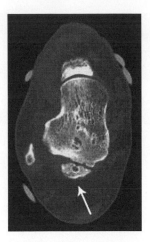

Fig. 2. Transversal CT scan of a 41-year-old male presenting with chronic right ankle pain on forced plantarflexion. At the age of 32, he sustained a supination, hyperplantarflexion trauma. The *arrow* indicates a symptomatic os trigonum. The subchondral sclerosis and cysts can be explained by the pathologic micromovement between os trigonum and talus.

present with anterior ankle pain, swelling after activity, and (slightly) limited dorsiflexion [4]. The diagnosis of anterior impingement is clinical, based on physical examination. Recognizable local pain on palpation is present anteriorly, and the osteophytes may be palpable with the ankle joint in slight plantarflexion.

A differentiation can be made between anteromedial and anterolateral impingement (Fig. 5). Patients are asked whether palpation of the anterior joint line reproduces the pain. Because the middle section is covered by neurovascular structures and tendons, this part of the joint is difficult to access by palpation. If a patient with a clinical anterior impingement syndrome experiences pain predominantly located anteromedially when palpated, the diagnosis is anteromedial impingement. If pain on palpation is predominantly located anterolaterally, the diagnosis is anterolateral impingement. Forced

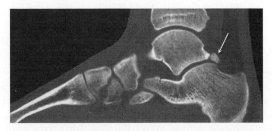

Fig. 3. Sagittal CT scan of the right ankle of a 30-year-old male professional soccer player. The patient presents with posterior ankle pain after a hyperplantarflexion trauma. The *arrow* indicates an os trigonum, which is slightly translocated to dorsal and inferior.

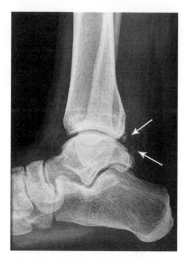

Fig. 4. Lateral X-ray of the left ankle of a 30-year-old male patient. During posterior arthroscopy multiple medially located bony calcifications were identified and removed. The *arrows* indicate these calcifications.

hyper dorsiflexion can provoke the pain, but this manoeuvrue can give false negative results.

Patients with posterior ankle impingement experience pain over the posterior aspect of the ankle joint, mainly on forced plantarflexion. In this position compression of soft tissue or bony structures between the posterior aspect of the distal tibia and calcaneus can occur. In some patients, forced dorsiflexion is also painful. In this dorsiflexed position, traction is applied to the posterior joint capsule and posterior talofibular ligament, both attaching to the posterior talar process.

On examination, there is pain on palpation of the posterior aspect of the talus. This posterior talar process can best be palpated posterolaterally between the peroneal tendons and the Achilles tendon (Fig. 6). Posteromedially, the neurovascular bundle and flexor tendons are covering the talus. Therefore, posteromedial pain on palpation does not automatically imply impingement. The passive forced plantarflexion test (Fig. 7) should be performed with repetitive quick passive hyperplantarflexion movements in a patient sitting with the knee flexed at 90°. The test can be repeated in slight external rotation or slight internal rotation of the foot on the tibia. The investigator can apply a rotational movement on the point of maximal plantarflexion, thereby "grinding" the posterior talar process/os trigonum between tibia and calcaneus. A negative test rules out a posterior impingement syndrome. A positive test, in combination with pain on posterolateral palpation, should be followed by a diagnostic infiltration. The infiltration is performed from the posterolateral side, making it possible to infiltrate the capsule with Xylocaine between the prominent posterior talar process and

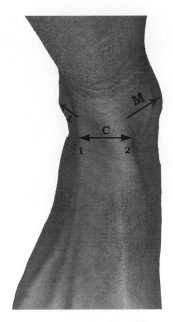

Fig. 5. Anterior view of a right ankle indicating the three different anterior regions. C is the central part of the joint, between the medial border of the anterior tibial tendon (indicated as 2) and the lateral border of the peroneus tertius tendon (indicated as 1). Medially of the central part, at the level of the joint line, is the anteromedial region as indicated with a M. Laterally of the central part, also at the level of the joint line, is the anterolateral region as indicated with a L.

the posterior edge of the tibia. If the pain on forced plantarflexion disappears, the diagnosis is confirmed.

Radiographic features

Standard anteroposterior and lateral radiographs are used to detect the presence of osteophytes [12]. In patients with anterior talar or tibial spurs, these are regarded as the cause of the anterior impingement syndrome. Due to their location, they lead to a "kissing" phenomena and concomitant pinching of hypertrophic synovial tissue. Because of the anteromedial notch [11], anteromedial osteophytes are not detected by standard radiographs in many patients with anterior impingement [20]. A cadaver study showed that anteromedial tibial osteophytes up to 7.3 mm in size, originating from the anteromedial border, remain undetected due to superposition or overprojection of the more prominent anterolateral border of the distal tibia [20]. Medially located talar osteophytes remain undetected due to over projection or superposition of the lateral part of the talar neck and body [20].

Detection of these osteophytes is important for preoperative planning. At surgery, differentiation between normal bony and soft tissue variants and pathologic conditions can be difficult, given subtle variations in joint

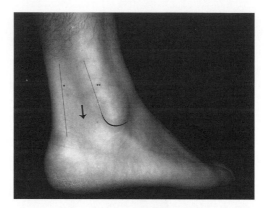

Fig. 6. Posterolateral view of right ankle indicating the region where the posterior talar process can be palpated. The region is located between the Achilles tendon (indicated with *) and the peroneal tendons (indicated with **). The *arrow* points at the location of the posterior talar process.

anatomy [27–29]. Especially in patients with accompanying synovial reflections, overlying the concealed osteophytes [28], anteromedial bony spurs are poorly visualized arthroscopically, and can therefore be missed easily. Radiographic classification of spur formation correlates with the surgical outcome [5,12,30]. An oblique radiograph evidences medially located tibial and talar osteophytes. In this oblique anteromedial impingement (AMI) view, the beam is tilted into a 45° craniocaudal direction with the leg in 30° of external rotation and the foot plantarflexed in relation to the standard lateral radiograph position (Fig. 8).

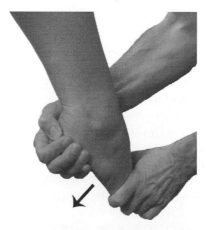

Fig. 7. The hyperplantarflexion test is performed in a sitting patient with the knee flexed in 90°. The foot is forced into maximal plantarflexion. In the case of the presence of a bony or soft tissue impediment this becomes impacted between the tibia and the calcaneus, leading to a sharp recognizable pain.

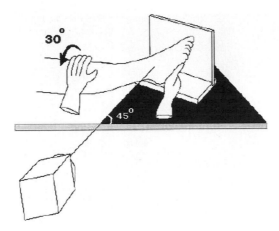

Fig. 8. Anteromedial impingement view (AMI) to detect anteromedial tibial and talar osteo-phytes. The beam is tilted into a 45° craniocaudal direction, while placing the leg in 30° exor-otation relative to the standard lateral radiograph position.

The sensitivity of lateral radiographs for detecting anterior tibial and ta-lar osteophytes is 40% and 32%, respectively (specificity 70% and 82%) [31]. When lateral radiographs are combined with oblique AMI radio-graphs, sensitivity increase to 85% for tibial and 73% for talar osteophytes. This increase is due to the high sensitivity of the oblique AMI radiographs for detecting anteromedial osteophytes (93% for tibial and 67% for talar os-teophytes). Standard lateral radiographs do not detect all anteriorly located osteophytes. Oblique AMI radiographs are a useful adjunct to routine ra-diographs, and recommended to detect anteromedial tibial and talar osteo-phytes (Fig. 9A–B).

In patients with posterior impingement, the anteroposterior (AP) ankle view typically does not show abnormalities. On the lateral view, a prominent posterior talar process or os trigonum can sometimes be recognized. The posterior talar process or os trigonum is located posterolaterally. This pos-terolateral part is often superimposed on the medial talar tubercle on the lateral radiographs. Therefore, detection of an os trigonum on a standard lateral view is often not possible. For the same reason, calcifications can sometimes not be detected by this standard lateral view. We recommend lat-eral radiographs with the foot in 25° of external rotation in relation to the standard lateral radiographs (Fig. 10A–B).

Especially following trauma, a CT scan can help to ascertain the extent of injury and exact location of calcifications or bony fragments.

Management and outcome

Conservative management, consisting of appropriately placed injections or heel lifts, is recommended in the early stages, but is frequently

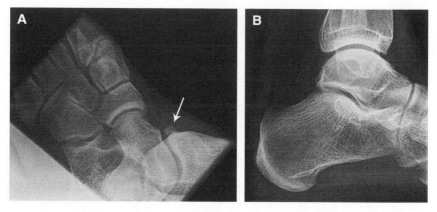

Fig. 9. Forty-three-year-old patient presenting with anteromedial left ankle pain during running. (*A*) Anteromedial impingement (AMI) view showing an osteophyte at the medial border of the distal tibia, as pointed out with the arrow. (*B*) In this standard lateral radiograph the medially located osteophyte on the anterior distal tibia remains undetected.

unsuccessful [4,8]. McMurray [2] reported the first surgically treated patients. Numerous authors have reported good results with open arthrotomy [14,32,33]. Open arthrotomy can be complicated by cutaneous nerve entrapment, damage of the long extensor tendons, wound dehiscence, and formation of hypertrophic scar tissue [4].

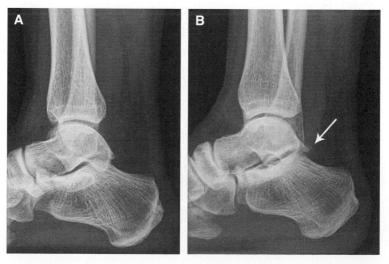

Fig. 10. Thirty-four-year-old male patient presenting with posterior right ankle pain during plantarflexion movements of the foot. (*A*) The standard lateral radiograph shows no abnormalities. (*B*) Lateral X-ray with the foot in 25° exorotation. A prominent posterior talar process including os trigonum can be recognized.

Before the advent of arthroscopy of the ankle joint, it was believed that this technique was unsuitable in view of the narrow joint space and convex talar anatomy [34].

At arthroscopy, patients are supine with slight elevation of the ipsilateral buttock. The heel of the affected foot rests on the very end of the operating table, thus making it possible for the surgeon to fully dorsiflex the ankle joint by leaning against the sole of the patient's foot. After making an ante-romedial skin incision, the subcutaneous layer is bluntly divided with a he-mostat (Fig. 11). A 4 mm, 30° angle arthroscope is used routinely. The anterolateral portal is made under arthroscopic control.

Osteophytes are removed using a 4-mm chisel or motorized shaver system (bone cutter or small acromioniser). These spurs can best be identified when the ankle is dorsiflexed. Distraction of the joint results in tightening of the anterior capsule, therefore making it more difficult to identify the osteo-phytes. Another advantage of the dorsiflexion position is that the talus is concealed in the joint, thereby protecting the weight bearing cartilage of the talus from potential iatrogenic damage. The contour of the anterior tibia is identified by shaving away the tissue just superior to the osteophyte

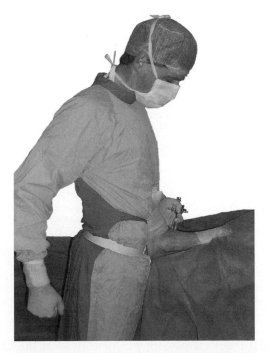

Fig. 11. Anterior ankle arthroscopy on a left ankle of a patient lying supine with the heel of the foot at the very end of the operating table. The medial portal is created with the foot in slight dorsal flexion by leaning of the surgeon to the sole of the foot. The trocard is introduced just medial of the anterior tibial tendon after having bluntly divided the vertical skin incision using a hemostat.

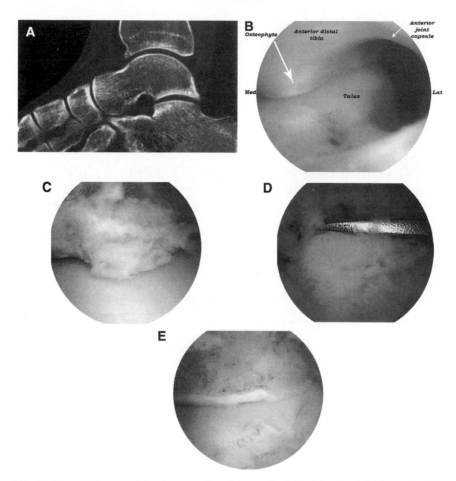

Fig. 12. Twenty-six-year-old male presenting with anterior left ankle pain. (*A*) The sagittal CT scan shows an osteophyte at the anterior distal tibia. (*B*) In this arthroscopic image the osteophyte is visualized as a prominence onto the distal tibia. The osteophyte is surrounded by scar tissue, and is therefore not clearly visible. By palpating the distal tibia by means of a probe, the osteophyte can be distinguished from the scar tissue attached to the distal tibia. (The arthroscope is introduced through the anteromedial portal). (*C*) Arthroscopic view through the same anteromedial portal after resection of the soft tissue medially, superiorly, and laterally of the osteophyte with a shaver. The osteophyte is clearly visible now. (*D*) The scope is still in the anteromedial portal, and the chisel is introduced through the anterolateral portal. The osteophyte is cleaved from the distal tibia by means of the chisel. (*E*) Arthroscopic image after removal of the osteophyte.

(Fig. 12 A–D). If there are osteophytes or ossicles at the tip of the medial malleolus, the medial malleolus is shaved generously after resection of the osteophyte (Fig. 13A–C).

Postoperative management involves a compression bandage and partial weight bearing for 3 to 5 days. Patients are instructed to actively dorsiflex

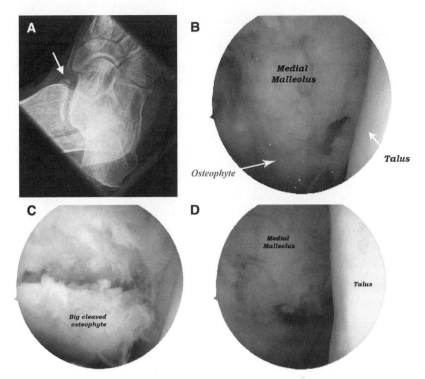

Fig. 13. Forty-eight-year-old male patient presenting with anterior medially located left ankle pain. (*A*) The anteromedial impingement view (AMI-view) reveals an osteophyte at the level of the medial malleolus, as indicated with the *arrow*. (*B*) The arthroscopic image shows osteophytes at the anterior edge and tip of the medial malleolus. The osteophytes are visualized through the scope positioned in the anterolateral portal. (*C*) The arthroscope is still in the anterolateral portal showing the cleaved osteophyte, performed by a chisel that was introduced through the anteromedial portal. (*D*) Postoperative arthroscopic image after removal of the osteophytes. The arthroscope is in the anterolateral portal showing the reduced medial malleolus.

their ankle and foot, and to repeat this exercise a few times every hour for the first 2 to 3 days after surgery [12].

From the late 1980s, several authors have published retrospective studies on management of anterior ankle impingement [3,16,35,36]. Good/excellent results varied between 57% and 67%, with an overall complication rate from 10% to 15%.

Ferkel reported on 31 patients with soft tissue impingement lesions [22], with a success rate of 84%. Comparable high percentages of good/excellent results, after arthroscopic management of synovial impingement lesions, were reported by others [5,37–39]. Less favorable results and a relative high percentage of (18%) temporary neurologic complications were reported [40]. Although there was a significant decrease in pain, only 26% of the patients reached their previous athletic activity level.

The first study with results of management for isolated anterior bony ankle impingement lesions was published by Ogilvie-Harris and colleagues [9]. At an average of 39 months follow-up (range 24–68 months) 15 of the 17 patients reported significant improvement. The complication rate was 18% (one superficial infection and two patients with residual numbness).

Scranton and McDermott [41] compared open and arthroscopic resection of impinging osteophytes [30]. Compared with an open procedure, patients undergoing arthroscopy recovered in approximately half the time and returned to full athletic training 1 month sooner. They also showed that the radiologic size and location of the osteophytes correlated with the outcome of surgery.

We prospectively documented the results of 62 consecutive patients with painful limited dorsiflexion of the ankle, not responding to conservative management. All 42 men and 20 women (average age 31 years) underwent arthroscopic surgery. Preoperative radiographs were graded according to an osteoarthritic and an impingement classification. Standardized follow-up took place at 4 months, 1 year, and 2 years after surgery. Results showed that the degree of osteoarthritic changes is a better prognostic factor for the outcome of arthroscopic surgery for anterior ankle impingement than spur size and location of the spurs. Osteophytes without joint space narrowing are not a manifestation of osteoarthric changes but rather the results of local (micro)trauma. After 2 years, 73% of the patients experienced overall excellent or good result; 90% of those without joint space narrowing had good or excellent results, and 50% of the patients with joint space narrowing had good or excellent results. At 2-year follow-up, the group without joint space narrowing showed significantly better scores in pain, swelling, ability to work, and involvement in sports. Our study also showed that patients with less than 2 years from ankle pain before surgery and with spurs located anteromedially were more satisfied than patients with longer periods of preoperative pain and with anterolateral spurs [12].

In 2001, we assessed a long-term follow-up on the same patient cohort [13]. In patients without joint space narrowing (grade 0 and grade I), the overall percentage of good/excellent results was 83%. For patients with joint space narrowing (grade II) the percentage of good/excellent results was still 53%. Asymptomatic osteophytes recurred in two-thirds of the ankles with grade I lesions. Coull and colleagues [42] reported recurrence of osteophytes in all their 27 patients who underwent open debridement. All patients with osteophyte recurrence had a history of ongoing supination trauma or repetitive forced dorsiflexion, most often as a result of regular participation in soccer. There was no statistical correlation between the recurrence of osteophytes and the return of symptoms. Cheng and Ferkel [43] found asymptomatic bony spurs in the ankles of 45% patients who played football and in 59% of patients who were dancers. Asymptomatic ankles may become painful after an injury [44].

All our patients with anterior osteophytic impingement had accompanying soft-tissue changes (synovitis or scar tissue). At arthroscopy, forced dorsiflexion produced impingement of the hypertrophic synovial tissue between the osteophytes. At follow-up, most ankles in which osteophytes had recurred were asymptomatic. It is not the osteophyte itself that is painful, but the compression of the synovial fold or fibrotic (scar) tissue causes pain.

There are a few descriptions about the arthroscopic management of the osteoarthritic ankle. Ogilvie-Harris and Sekyi-Out [9] used a subjective and functional scoring system to define successful management. At a mean follow-up of 45 months, there were only a few excellent or good results. However, 63% of the patients reported marked improvement and were satisfied with the procedure. These favorable results are supported by some authors [43], and denied by others [3,36,45]. Patient satisfaction was good/excellent in 53% of our patients with grade II osteoarthritic changes at an average of 6.5 years after surgery (5–8 years).

In our series, apart from three patients who needed additional surgery, all patients with grade II lesions (osteophytes with joint space narrowing) still had less pain at long-term follow-up. Approximately half of them rated satisfaction from good to excellent. In most ankles, narrowing of the joint space had not progressed. Given that the alternative is arthrodesis, these results are acceptable. Nevertheless, patients should be informed about the limitations of the procedure and chance of additional surgery.

Hamilton and colleagues [24] reported a good or excellent result in 30/40 (75%) open operations for posterior impingement syndrome and flexor hallucis longus tendinopathy at the expense of 15% complications. Marotta and colleagues [46] studied 12 patients with 17% complications. Full-performance dancing was possible at a mean of 3 months, with sporadic pain in 67% of the cases. In dancers, sport resumption has been reported to take place after 13 to 25 weeks [9,19]. Abramowitz and colleagues describe the result of operative management in 41 patients with posterior impingement [47]. Overall, full recovery time averaged 5 months. Complications occurred in 10 of 41 patients (24%) and average postoperative American Orthopaedic Foot and Ankle Society (AOFAS) score was 87.6%.

Between April 1994 and August 2000, we prospectively documented 57 consecutive patients with posterior ankle pain with a painful limitation on plantar flexion. Based on the radiographs, and including CT scanning, a distinction was made between bony and soft-tissue impingement. Endoscopic surgery was performed as an outpatient procedure in all patients.

Surgical technique for posterior ankle impingement

The patient is placed prone. The posterolateral portal is made at the level or slightly above the tip of the lateral malleolus, just lateral to the Achilles tendon (Fig. 14). After a vertical skin incision the subcutaneous layer is split by a mosquito clamp. The mosquito clamp is directed toward the interdigital webspace between first and second toe (Fig. 15). The mosquito clamp is

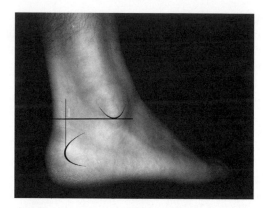

Fig. 14. Location of the posterolateral portal. The tip of the lateral malleolus, the distal lateral part of the Achilles tendon, as well as the contour of the calcaneus are marked onto the skin with black lines. A line is drawn parallel to the sole of the foot through the tip of the lateral malleolus. Just superior to the position where this line crosses the line that indicates the anterior part of the Achilles tendon, the posterolateral portal is situated (indicated with the white vertical line).

exchanged for the 4-mm arthroscope shaft with a blunt trocard, pointing into the same direction. Next, the posteromedial portal is made just medially of the Achilles tendon, in the horizontal plane at the same level as the posterolateral portal (Fig. 16). After making a vertical skin incision, the mosquito clamp is pointed into the direction of the arthroscopic shaft (already in place through the posterolateral portal). When the mosquito clamp touches the arthroscopic shaft, the shaft is used as a guide to "travel" into the direction of the ankle joint. The arthroscopic shaft is subsequently pulled slightly backward until the tip of the mosquito clamp becomes visible. The soft tissue just in front of the arthroscopic tip is spread with the mosquito clamp. After exchanging the mosquito clamp for a 5-mm full-radius resector, the fatty tissue overlying the posterior ankle capsule, lateral from the flexor hallucis longus tendon, is resected. The procedure typically starts on the lateral side at the level of the subtalar joint. The ankle or subtalar joint can be entered easily by opening the very thin joint capsule. The operation typically involves removal of the hypertrophic posterior joint capsule, removal of an os trigonum or a hypertrophic posterior talar process and release of the flexor hallucis longus (Fig. 17 A–D). After surgery, patients are instructed to weight bear as tolerated.

Results

Sixty-three procedures were performed in 57 patients, with a mean postoperative follow-up of 38 months (range 24–54 months). No patient was lost in follow-up. A single complication consisted of temporary loss of sensation

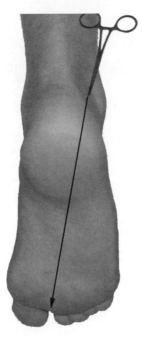

Fig. 15. After creating the posterolateral portal, as explained in Fig. 14, the subcutaneous skin is split with a mosquito clamp that must be directed toward the interdigital webspace between the first and second toe (as indicated with the black line).

of the posteromedial heel in one patient. Overall return to work was 3 weeks (range 1–8 weeks), return to sports activities took place at an average of nine weeks (range 2 52 weeks). The overall percentage of good/excellent results was 80%.

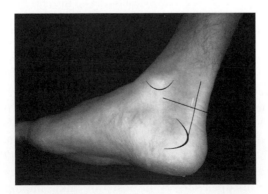

Fig. 16. Location of the posteromedial portal. The medial malleolus, the medial distal part of the calcaneus, as well as the contour of the calcaneus, are marked onto the skin in black. A horizontal line drawn parallel to the sole of the foot, just inferior of the lateral malleolus, is drawn in black over the Achilles tendon to medial. The posteromedial portal (indicated with the white vertical line) is located at the level just medial to the Achilles tendon, at the same level as the posterolateral portal.

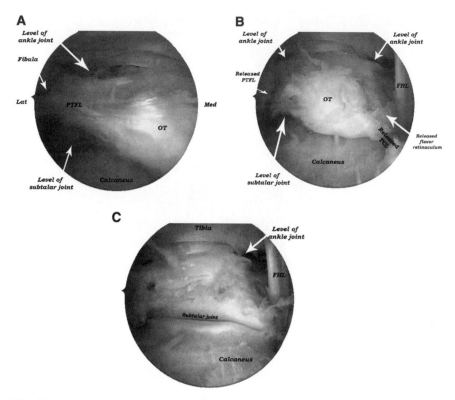

Fig. 17. Forty-four-year-old patient presenting with posterior left ankle pain for 3 years, which progressed over the last year. The X-ray revealed an os trigonum as a cause of the pain. (*A*) Endoscopic view of the posterior aspect of the left ankle. The connection of the os trigonum (OT) with the posterior talofibular ligament (PTFL) is clearly visualized with the arthroscope in the posterolateral portal. (*B*) The os trigonum is released from the PTFL, the talocalcaneal ligament (TCL), as well as from its connection with the Flexor Hallucis Longus (FHL) retinaculum using a punch introduced via the posteromedial portal. (*C*) The arthroscope is in the posterolateral portal. The os trigonum has been removed by means of a small chisel and grasper.

Our results compare favorably with the results of open surgery. In the combined posttraumatic and overuse group, we found an average recovery time to sports activities of 9 weeks, compared with 13 to 25 weeks in the patients undergoing open surgery [10,19]. Our complication rate compares favorably with the 9% complications rate stated by Ferkel [22] occurring in foot and ankle arthroscopy in general, and with the complication rate found in the literature for open surgery in posterior ankle impingement, ranging from 15% to 24% [24,46–48].

The use of an anterolateral portal, combined with a posterolateral or subtalar portal, is an alternative to approach the posterior compartment of the ankle joint. When combined with anterior ankle arthroscopy, most surgeons regard the posteromedial portal to be contraindicated in all but the most extreme situations, because of the potential of serious complications. The posterolateral portal, however, is used routinely by most authors.

For management of posterior ankle impingement the two-portal posterior endoscopic ankle approach with the patient in a prone position has shown to offer excellent access to the posterior compartment of the ankle joint, the posterior subtalar joint, the flexor hallucis longus tendon, and os trigonum.

Overuse patients do better than patients with impingement after a traumatic event. Return to work and sports activities was faster in patients treated for overuse than for posttraumatic causes. The better outcome in patients with an overuse syndrome can partly be explained by the additional injuries to the ankle structures in patients with posttraumatic impingement syndrome. This additional pathology is most likely the reason for residual complaints in these patients [41]. Patients arthroscoped for bony impingement did better than patients arthroscoped for soft-tissue impingement. Misdiagnosis in soft-tissue impingement is more likely to occur compared with bony impingement. Furthermore, recurrence of scar tissue postoperatively is another potential reason for failure.

Management of posterior ankle impingement, by means of a two-portal endoscopic hindfoot approach, compares favorably to open surgery. Hindfoot endoscopy causes less morbidity and facilitates a quick recovery. It is recommended that the procedure is performed by an experienced arthroscopist, who has studied the local anatomy in a cadaveric setting.

Acknowledgment

Many thanks are given to P.A.J. de Leeuw, PhD fellow, for recording and editing the arthroscopic/endoscopic images.

References

[1] Morris LH. Report of cases of athlete's ankle. J Bone Joint Surg 1943;25:220–4.

[2] Mc Murray TP. Footballer's ankle. J Bone Joint Surg 1950;32:68–9.

[3] Biedert R. Anterior ankle pain in sports medicine: aetiology and indications for arthroscopy. Arch Orthop Trauma Surg 1991;110:293–7.

[4] Cutsuries AM, Saltrick KR, Wagner J, et al. Arthroscopic arthroplasty of the ankle joint. Clin Podiatr Med Surg 1994;11:449–67.

[5] Ferkel RD, Fasulo GJ. Arthroscopic treatment of ankle injuries. Orthop Clin North Am 1994;25:17–32.

[6] Hermodsson I. The development of coxarthrosis. A radiological follow-up of patients operated upon. Radiologe 1983;23:378–84.

[7] van Dijk CN, Lim LS, Poortman A, et al. Degenerative joint disease in female ballet dancers. Am J Sports Med 1995;23:295–300.

[8] Ferkel RD, Scranton PE Jr. Arthroscopy of the ankle and foot. J Bone Joint Surg Am 1993; 75:1233–42.

[9] Ogilvie-Harris DJ, Mahomed N, Demaziere A. Anterior impingement of the ankle treated by arthroscopic removal of bony spurs. J Bone Joint Surg Br 1993;75:437–40.

[10] Handoll HH, Rowe BH, Quinn KM, et al. Interventions for preventing ankle ligament injuries. Cochrane Database Syst Rev 2001:CD000018.

[11] Tol JL, van Dijk CN. Etiology of the anterior ankle impingement syndrome: a descriptive anatomical study. Foot Ankle Int 2004;25:382–6.

[12] van Dijk CN, Tol JL, Verheyen CC. A prospective study of prognostic factors concerning the outcome of arthroscopic surgery for anterior ankle impingement. Am J Sports Med 1997;25: 737–45.

[13] Tol JL, Verheyen CP, van Dijk CN. Arthroscopic treatment of anterior impingement in the ankle. J Bone Joint Surg Br 2001;83:9–13.

[14] O'Donoghue DH. Impingement exostoses of the talus and tibia. J Bone Joint Surg Am 1957; 39-A:835–52.

[15] Williams JM, Brandt KD. Exercise increases osteophyte formation and diminishes fibrillation following chemically induced articular cartilage injury. J Anat 1984;139(Pt 4):599–611.

[16] Hawkins RB. Arthroscopic treatment of sports-related anterior osteophytes in the ankle. Foot Ankle 1988;9:87–90.

[17] van Dijk CN. On diagnostic strategies in patients with severe ankle sprain. Amsterdam: University of Amsterdam; 1994.

[18] van Dijk CN, Bossuyt PM, Marti RK. Medial ankle pain after lateral ligament rupture. J Bone Joint Surg Br 1996;78:562–7.

[19] Krips R, van Dijk CN, Halasi T, et al. Anatomical reconstruction versus tenodesis for the treatment of chronic anterolateral instability of the ankle joint: a 2- to 10-year follow-up, multicenter study. Knee Surg Sports Traumatol Arthrosc 2000;8:173–9.

[20] Tol JL, Slim E, van Soest AJ, et al. The relationship of the kicking action in soccer and anterior ankle impingement syndrome. A biomechanical analysis. Am J Sports Med 2002;30: 45–50.

[21] Berberian WS, Hecht PJ, Wapner KL, et al. Morphology of tibiotalar osteophytes in anterior ankle impingement. Foot Ankle Int 2001;22:313–7.

[22] Ferkel RD, Karzel RP, Del Pizzo W, et al. Arthroscopic treatment of anterolateral impingement of the ankle. Am J Sports Med 1991;19:440–6.

[23] Stibbe AB, Van Dijk CN, Marti RK. The os trigonum syndrome. Acta Orthop Scand 1994;(Suppl 262):59–60.

[24] Hamilton WG, Geppert MJ, Thompson FM. Pain in the posterior aspect of the ankle in dancers. Differential diagnosis and operative treatment. J Bone Joint Surg Am 1996;78: 1491–500.

[25] Hedrick MR, McBryde AM. Posterior ankle impingement. Foot Ankle Int 1994;15:2–8.

[26] St Pierre RK, Velazco A, Fleming LL. Impingement exostoses of the talus and fibula secondary to an inversion sprain. A case report. Foot Ankle 1983;3:282–5.

[27] Ferkel RD. Chapter 2. In: Wipple TL, editor. Arthroscopic surgery: the foot and the ankle. Philadelphia: Lippincott-Raven Publishers; 1996. p. 13–46.

[28] Ray RG, Gusman DN, Christensen JC. Anatomical variation of the tibial plafond: the anteromedial tibial notch. J Foot Ankle Surg 1994;33:419–26.

[29] Vogler HW, Stienstra JJ, Montgomery F, et al. Anterior ankle impingement arthropathy. The role of anterolateral arthrotomy and arthroscopy. Clin Podiatr Med Surg 1994;11:425–47.

[30] Scranton PE Jr, McDermott JE. Anterior tibiotalar spurs: a comparison of open versus arthroscopic debridement. Foot Ankle 1992;13:125–9.

[31] Tol JL, Verhagen RA, Krips R, et al. The anterior ankle impingement syndrome: diagnostic value of oblique radiographs. Foot Ankle Int 2004;25:63–8.

[32] Hensley JP, Saltrick K, Le T. Anterior ankle arthroplasty: a retrospective study. J Foot Surg 1990;29:169–72.

[33] Parkes JC, Hamilton WG, Patterson AH, et al. The anterior impingement syndrome of the ankle. J Trauma 1980;20:895–8.

[34] Burman MS. Arthroscopy of direct visualization of joints. An experimental cadaver study. J Bone Joint Surg 2006;13:669–95.

[35] Feder KS, Schonholtz GJ. Ankle arthroscopy: review and long-term results. Foot Ankle 1992;13:382–5.
[36] Martin DF, Baker CL, Curl WW, et al. Operative ankle arthroscopy. Long-term followup. Am J Sports Med 1989;17:16–23.
[37] Clasper JC, Pailthorpe CA. Chronic ankle pain in soldiers: the role of ankle arthroscopy and soft tissue excision. J R Army Med Corps 1996;142:107–9.
[38] Meislin RJ, Rose DJ, Parisien JS, et al. Arthroscopic treatment of synovial impingement of the ankle. Am J Sports Med 1993;21:186–9.
[39] Thein R, Eichenblat M. Arthroscopic treatment of sports-related synovitis of the ankle. Am J Sports Med 1992;20:496–8.
[40] Jerosch J, Steinbeck J, Schneider T, et al. Arthroscopic treatment of anterior synovitis of the upper ankle joint in the athlete. Sportverletz Sportschaden 1994;8:67–72.
[41] Scranton PE Jr, McDermott JE. Anterior tibiotalar spurs: a comparison of open versus arthroscopic debridement. Foot Ankle 1992;13:125–9.
[42] Coull R, Raffiq T, James LE, et al. Open treatment of anterior impingement of the ankle. J Bone Joint Surg Br 2003;85:550–3.
[43] Cheng JC, Ferkel RD. The role of arthroscopy in ankle and subtalar degenerative joint disease. Clin Orthop Relat Res 1998;65–72.
[44] van Dijk CN, Verhagen RA, Tol JL. Arthroscopy for problems after ankle fracture. J Bone Joint Surg Br 1997;79:280–4.
[45] Cerulli G, Caraffa A, Buompadre V, et al. Operative arthroscopy of the ankle. Arthroscopy 1992;8:537–40.
[46] Marotta JJ, Micheli LJ. Os trigonum impingement in dancers. Am J Sports Med 1992;20: 533–6.
[47] Abramowitz Y, Wollstein R, Barzilay Y, et al. Outcome of resection of a symptomatic os trigonum. J Bone Joint Surg Am 2003;85-A:1051–7.
[48] Callanan I, Williams L, Stephens M. "Os post peronei" and the posterolateral nutcracker impingement syndrome. Foot Ankle Int 1998;19:475–8.

**ELSEVIER
SAUNDERS**

Foot Ankle Clin N Am
11 (2006) 685–701

**FOOT AND
ANKLE CLINICS**

Index

Note: Page numbers of article titles are in **boldface** type.

1083-7515/06/$ - see front matter © 2006 Elsevier Inc. All rights reserved.
doi:10.1016/S1083-7515(06)00079-9

Moving?

Make sure your subscription moves with you!

To notify us of your new address, find your **Clinics Account Number** (located on your mailing label above your name), and contact customer service at:

E-mail: elspcs@elsevier.com

800-654-2452 (subscribers in the U.S. & Canada)
407-345-4000 (subscribers outside of the U.S. & Canada)

Fax number: 407-363-9661

Elsevier Periodicals Customer Service
6277 Sea Harbor Drive
Orlando, FL 32887-4800

*To ensure uninterrupted delivery of your subscription, please notify us at least 4 weeks in advance of move.